FOOD:
YOU'RE THE
BOSS!
PUT IT TO WORK FOR YOU

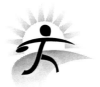

FOOD: YOU'RE THE BOSS!

PUT IT TO WORK FOR YOU

Five Steps to Building
Your Nutrition Success

Gary R. Epler, M.D.

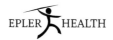

Epler, Gary R.

Food: You're the Boss
Put It to Work for You

Library of Congress Control Number: 2012908063
ISBN: 978-0-9849335-3-2

Printed in the United States of America

Other books by Gary Epler:
You're the Boss: Manage Your Disease
BOOP: You're the Boss
Asthma: You're the Boss

*This book is dedicated to people everywhere
who manage their nutrition successfully.*

Acknowledgments

I would like to thank Marc David for his phenomenal insight into nutrition management and his extraordinary help. I would also like to thank Roberta Anding for her nutritional information, teachings, and food safety issues—"If in doubt, throw it out." I wish to give a special thanks to Chef German Lam for his creative nutritional ingenuity and healthy cooking with "swagger." Thanks also to Glenda Garland for her wonderful writing assistance, to Steve Cumming for his outstanding editing and title development, and to Marian Ferro for her unerring proofreading.

Contents

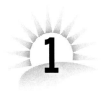

Food is Your Friend:
Make It Work for You with Five Steps

You are in charge of your nutrition. You can manage it better than anyone else. Use the following five key steps for success:

- Learn everything you can about nutrition.
- Understand your nutritional inventory and the diagnostic process.
- Know your options for nutrition management.
- Monitor your nutritional status.
- Create a lifetime environment for maintaining nutritional health.

This chapter will provide you with a general approach to managing your nutrition. Specific strategies will be discussed in the chapters that follow.

Begin the process by understanding that you need to take a positive approach to your nutrition.

Food is not an enemy. It's your friend. It provides you with energy and nutrients for a life filled with creativity and excitement. You just need to know what, when, how, and where to eat. Learn to use nutrition that will provide high-level energy by eating the right amount of high-quality foods at the right time.

The traditional approach to nutrition management has been to find solutions utilizing pills and popular diets. These approaches can be helpful for some people. But, too often they can lead to confusion, dangerous results, and no long-term solutions.

Healthy metabolism depends on complex physical and mind interactions that are capable of changing rapidly.

The successful approach involves actively taking charge. Manage your nutrition by learning everything you can about nutrition and about your management options, monitoring your progress, and creating a healing environment for long-term success.

Learn about metabolism of carbohydrates and fat. Learn about the carbohydrate and fat danger threshold levels. Some carbs—the bad-quantity carbs—have low thresholds; small amounts trigger weight gain and vascular inflammation. Some fats—the bad-quantity fats—have low thresholds; small amounts cause cellular inflammation leading to heart disease and strokes.

Good carbs are vegetables like spinach, fruits, and legumes like peas and beans. Bad-quantity carbs are sugar, sugary foods and drinks, refined grains, and processed carbs like pastries, candy, chips, and fried potatoes.

Good fats are the unsaturated fats like omega-3 foods and olive oil. Bad-quantity fats are the saturated fats like meat fat and lard.

————

Olivia Fenston became obsessed about losing weight. She had gained 20 pounds during her college years and had not found a way to lose them.

She tried pills.

"Take one of these capsules and one of these tablets each morning," her doctor had told her. The doctor also had explained in detail the potential side effects, and warned her about one potentially life-threatening effect, but she apparently wasn't listening. She had weight to lose and the pills were going to help.

She thought that everyone else was thin and beautiful, and she had to be the same way or she couldn't enjoy life. Yes, it was irrational and she knew it, but she didn't care. She had weight to lose.

"Look at the weight I'm losing," Olivia said to herself excitedly two weeks after starting on the pills. She had lost 15 pounds. "This is fantastic," she thought. "I'm going to be thin and beautiful."

Shortly afterward, however, she panicked when she felt a sharp pain in her right side just above the liver. She had heard about someone who had taken the same pills and had developed a severe side effect that required a lung transplantation.

She rushed to see her doctor.

"Let's see what going on," the doctor said calmly. "It's probably a diaphragmatic muscle pull and not related to the pills."

"I don't care what it is," Olivia said frantically. "I'm not taking those pills. They'll kill me."

"That's a wise decision," the doctor said. "You look perfect just the way you are."

The doctor was right. We are all perfect just the way we are, but she didn't believe it and had to lose weight regardless of the dangers.

So Olivia started a vegetarian diet. However she failed to take the time to learn about the need for protein or to create a healthy diet plan. She believed that if she didn't consume meat or fish, she'd lose weight.

Two weeks later, she was cranky and irritable. She annoyed her friends by incessantly telling everyone about her diet, and she had gained two pounds. By three months, she was more frustrated than ever. Olivia had gained ten pounds! She also had a weakened immune system with inflamed skin lesions and prolonged recovery from colds.

How is this possible? It was obvious to everyone else. She had been eating pasta, cheese, and salads, and was stressed to the maximum.

These foods turn into storage fat, increasing weight. The stress triggered cortisol, which is a glucocorticoid steroid released by the adrenal glands, causing excessive blood sugar that is converted to abdominal fat.

Olivia was desperate. She hadn't lost weight from her previous gain of two pounds, and now she had gained another ten pounds.

She then heard about a miracle weight-loss guava juice that was made with a leafy vegetable grown in Southeast Asia. It was from an exotic location and it was natural, so it had to work, she thought.

"Stop! Don't take that drink," Olivia's friend said.

"Why not?"

"It can cause constrictive bronchiolitis."

"What? What'd you say?" Olivia asked. "I can't even pronounce it."

"That drink can cause some rare lung disease by scarring the small airways and can even cause death in really bad situations," her friend answered. "It was banned in Southeast Asia."

"That's impossible. How can vegetable leaves cause a problem with the lungs?"

"It contains a toxin that attacks the airways."

"I'm glad you told me. Forget it. I'm not touching that drink."

So, Olivia signed up for a weight-loss spa program advertised on television. The instructors taught her about metabolism and healthy nutrition, which was good, but she didn't really absorb any of the information. The spa program also included an exercise program, but to Olivia, it was too much work.

She attended a mind-body institute weight-loss program, but it didn't work for her because she kept falling asleep.

Meanwhile, Olivia was so stressed about trying to lose weight that she gained another ten pounds.

Several years later, Olivia had failed to find the right program and reached the obesity range. She developed diabetes and hypertension, and continued to feel that everyone was so thin and beautiful and that she wasn't. She developed severe depression and lost her job.

———

Unfortunately, similar sad stories are repeated too often among people all over the world. People feel they must lose weight, whether it's 20 pounds or 100 pounds, and obsession takes over their lives. They search for pills, for diets, for anything that will easily make the weight go away, failing to realize that they're the solution by actively developing a successful lifelong program.

Nutrition is a complex system that combines the mind and the body. The process of developing a program begins with learning everything possible about nutrition.

———

Wendy Martin gained 20 pounds during her college years, but really didn't pay attention to the gain and had no feelings about trying to look thin or beautiful like the women in magazines and on television

She felt good about herself, but realized her flabby belly wasn't attractive and decided to eliminate it. She had only gained 20 pounds, but realized that it may take two years to lose it and that it wouldn't be an easy, one-step fix.

Wendy began with the first step: She learned about nutrition. She bought an audiobook and listened to it during her 30-minute drive to work. She visited internet sites and learned about carbohydrate metabolism and abdominal fat. She learned about fat and protein metabolism, and vitamins and minerals. She even learned about water and hydration.

Wendy had heard about the dangers of diet pills, and after studying the different types, concluded that some of them were effective in the short term but the potential side effects were not worth the risk.

"How should I approach the situation?" Wendy asked a sports nutritionist.

"First, continue your positive approach and keep learning," the nutritionist said. "You have developed a good beginning by approaching nutrition with an attitude that will lead to success.

"Second step, let's take a nutrition inventory."

Wendy recorded her height and weight. From these two values, she calculated her body mass index, or BMI, which was 28.5—not too high but above the normal level of 25. She measured her waist circumference, and calculated her body fat percentage, which was 22%—again, not too high, but also above the healthy level.

Wendy and her nutritionist calculated how many calories and the volume of water she needed on a daily basis. To complete the inventory, her blood pressure, her fasting blood sugar, and her kidney function were measured as baselines to ensure that she had not developed early signs of excessive weight-related medical conditions such as diabetes or hypertension.

"This is great," Wendy said. "I really know where I stand, and I now have a basis to go forward."

"That's the second step," the nutritionist said. "Now, let's look at the third step—the management options."

"I've read about diet pills," Wendy said. "There seem to be different types. Some suppress appetite. Some ramp up the body to burn extra calories. Some claim to manipulate hormones. But none are for me. They have too many potentially dangerous side effects, and they're not permanent solutions."

"Let's talk about diets," the nutritionist said. "There are millions of them."

"I found out they're like pills in some ways," Wendy said. "Follow a list of specific foods. But they do have some good components, such as low saturated fat, low sugar, low sodium, or high fiber. They can help some people. For me, they're too complicated and not a lifetime solution because foods change over time and our metabolism efficiency changes over time."

"You've done your homework. Specific diets for diseases can be very useful short term, but we're talking long term."

"So," Wendy said, "now that we've discussed pills and diets, what's left?"

"You develop a nutrition plan that's best for you," the nutritionist said. "It's the what, when, how, and where answers that work."

Wendy learned the answers to these questions that were right for her. She used her personal nutrition monitors and soon returned to her healthy weight, which enriched her enthusiasm and energy.

She understood her nutrition, ate healthy foods in the right amounts at the right times and in the right places.

———

We have two stories, each of which tells us about 20 extra pounds. Does either one apply to you?

Olivia is a wonderful person but did everything wrong. She became obsessed about losing weight. She failed to learn about nutrition. She failed to learn about her body's nutritional status. She hoped that pills and diets would lead to a solution, but didn't know that she was so stressed out from wanting to lose weight that, paradoxically, these methods didn't work because the stress released more cortisol, creating increased fat storage. Importantly, she wasn't being herself. She wanted to be someone else—a thin person she saw in magazines and on TV.

Wendy did it correctly. She approached her weight loss in a positive manner. She learned about nutrition. She asked questions and understood the answers. She took a nutritional inventory. Wendy took charge of her nutrition and found a solution.

How can you take charge of your nutrition?

Follow the five vital steps. Begin with the first one: **Learn everything you can about nutrition.**

Ask your doctor and nutritionist, but don't stop there. Read books. Read reports and scientific studies. Follow Wendy's example. Listen to an audiobook or seminar in your car. Explore the internet to discover the best websites for you. Join discussion groups on the social media sites. You'll find people all over the world who have similar questions and concerns. They're just like you. They're learning to take charge and manage their nutrition.

———

Dave and Kelly were talking about diets and food during their lunch break. "I need your advice," Dave said. "I've got to lose this extra 20 pounds around my belly. What should I do?"

"Whoa, you're asking me?" Kelly asked jokingly.

"Yup. You look trim and healthy, so I'm sure you can help me. I've tried pills and diets. The pills are too dangerous. The diets are too confusing and too many rules, and I was annoying everyone and myself by always talking about being on a diet. Besides, I couldn't follow any of them long enough to help. What'd you do?"

"It's hard work," Kelly said, "but not impossible. I put in the work and the food works for me. I learned everything I could about nutrition. This is what I found: eat the right food in the right amount at the right time, and it'll take care of you forever!"

"That sounds exciting. But what do you mean?"

"Eat the right foods—carbohydrates like vegetables, fruit, whole grains, and fiber, fats like omega-3 foods, and lean protein," Kelly said. "Eat the right amount, too—learn the food thresholds. All foods are good. It's going over the threshold amount that's bad—eat over the threshold and some foods will cause inflamed arteries and fat bellies."

"What's a food threshold?" Dave asked.

"At a certain low level no food is dangerous, even the toxic puffer fish, but above that level, that puffer fish can kill you," Kelly said dramatically. "Many types of common carbohydrates and foods containing saturated fats have low threshold levels, especially processed foods and sugary drinks. Try eating one french fry or one potato chip, or one sip of a smoothie?" Kelly shook her head. "It's so easy to go over the risk threshold with these foods that I just try to avoid them most days, and that strategy works for me. Fortunately, there are many healthy foods—like spinach, vegetables, and omega-3 foods—that have such high thresholds you can eat much more of them and be safe."

"So, you're saying to keep healthy," Dave said, "I should eat the right foods in the right amounts, and they will protect my blood vessels, my heart, and provide the high energy I need to have an exciting, productive day."

"You got it! That's it," Kelly said as they returned to work.

———

After you've learned about nutrition, follow the second step: **Understand your nutritional inventory and the diagnostic process.**

Take a nutritional inventory. Begin with your height and weight. Calculate your body mass index (BMI). Measure your waist circumference. Determine your body fat percentage—it'll tell you about your lean muscle mass.

The major overweight diseases include hypertension, diabetes, and cardiovascular disease, as well as the complications of these disorders such as heart disease, stroke, kidney disease, eye disease, and arterial vascular disease.

The diagnostic process has three components. The first is an organized series of questions designed to lead to the diagnosis. The second is the physical examination. The third is a sequential group of diagnostic tests and procedures. The first two components require your close attention. It's the third that requires your active participation so that you can make decisions that are best for you.

Let's discuss the third step: **Know your management and treatment options.**

There are always options. Each situation is unique, and one option will be best for you.

You can explore diet pills, and be sure to ask about effectiveness. If you like statistics, get the numbers. Importantly, ask about the short-term risks and especially the long-term risks in terms of five to ten years, or even longer. What are the alternatives?

You can explore diet programs. Find out about the long-term effectiveness and about the risks. Each of these diet plans has associated risks.

You can explore surgical treatments, but you would be entering into potentially serious risks. It's important to find out the effectiveness –again the long-term effectiveness in terms of ten and 20 years. Find out about the risks—short-term, including anesthesia and the first 24 hours after surgery—and the long-term risks during the first five years and at 20 years?

You can explore organized weight-loss programs. Find out about the details of the methods used. Find out about the long-term effectiveness of these methods. What are the costs, including follow-up costs? Risks may not be listed in the brochure or website, but ask about short-term risks that may occur during the program, and the long-term risks as well.

The next step is to follow the fourth vital rule: **Monitor your nutritional status.**

Recording your weight is probably the most traditional and simple monitor. Daily weigh-ins are helpful in the hospital setting and for monitoring congestive heart failure, but long-term monitoring is needed for weight loss. During the initial few days, almost all options will result in weight loss, either from losing water weight or from consuming fewer calories.

Body fat percentage is a useful nutritional monitor because it reflects lean body mass, and lower numbers are good. People's weight may be at the high normal range, but they could be classified as metabolic obese if the body fat percentage is high, which results in increased risk for diabetes and hypertension.

The waist circumference at the belly button is an excellent nutritional monitor because it's easy, and decreasing the measurement to healthy levels will decrease the risk of developing overweight complications such as cardiovascular disease and diabetes.

You have now reached the final process for nutrition management. Use the fifth vital step: **Create a lifelong healing environment in which to manage your nutrition.**

Your body has an almost unlimited ability to manage its nutritional status. You have to know how to let this happen, as the ability may be dormant or blunted by the intensity of daily life. Use the power of the mind and the physical aspects of exercise and sleep.

First, use a positive approach. Say to yourself that you can successfully manage your situation. This will allow you to have more energy, follow your nutrition program, and take control. Remember, foods can provide boundless energy; it's the combination of how much, when, why, and where that's important.

Approaching nutrition in a positive manner will also help you to avoid the neurolinguistic trap. Neurolinguistics is the connection between your words and your actions. If you continually say negative words, eventually you'll establish harmful thinking pathways that, over time, change how you act and who you are.

This can occur in a weight-loss program. If you constantly use phrases such as "I can't lose weight," "I always gain weight no matter what," and "Nothing works for me" to describe your problems with weight, you create a pathway in your brain so ingrained that it's impossible to lose weight.

The solution is to build a neuropathway bypass to override the dysfunctional pathway by avoiding the negative words and substituting beneficial phrases, such as "There are solutions," "I can attain my healthy weight," and "This plan will work."

Use visualization: Visualize your healthy weight. Every cell in the body is continuously replaced, some every few minutes and others every few weeks or months. Visualize healthy, strong cells with no excess fat.

You can use this visualization process three or four times each day or any time you wish.

Use compassion: You're perfect the way you are. Give yourself compassion and give compassion to all of your organ systems. This concept is a little unusual, but strangely enough, it's comforting and gives you energy. Compassion is an excellent word. Some Tibetan monks live their entire lives meditating about compassion. People in their presence feel love and peace even without talking to them or touching them.

Use controlled breathing. This method has been around for years; anyone who has attended pregnancy classes knows the power of breathing. During a quiet time, breathe in 50% of your breath and breathe out 50%. Concentrate on taking equal breaths—the same amount in and out. During this breathing procedure, another option is to visualize breathing in healing energy that will spread throughout the entire body, providing energy by which you can succeed with your nutritional program. It's calming. It will create a strong nutrition-management environment.

Be persistent, as these methods require repetition and time—often weeks, months, or years. Our bodies have an endless energy-based system that can be used to create powerful changes and improve our lives.

The traditional sciences have two additional potent tools that help us create an environment in which to succeed with our nutritional program: a routine exercise program and a good sleep-hygiene program.

An exercise program that includes aerobic and muscle training can be a phenomenal component of your nutritional program. Begin slowly with a few minutes every other day, and advance to 45 minutes to an hour three to five or even seven times each week. Strength training should be part of your exercise program because it can diminish the loss of lean body mass.

Exercise will improve conditioning. It will improve the efficient use of oxygen by your muscles. And, importantly, it will improve your sense of well-being. You will feel that you're in control of the situation.

Sleep also can help create a successful nutritional program. Years of study have indicated that eight hours of sleep daily appears to be a requirement for a healthy life. Most people don't get enough sleep.

A healthy sleep-hygiene program consists of not allowing yourself to fall asleep watching television before you go to bed, not eating or eating very little within at least three hours before you go to sleep, and going to bed and waking up eight hours later regularly every night.

Managing sleep successfully can have a profound influence on your nutritional program.

———

Kate's a hero and let's find out why. She is in her 30s and enjoys time with her two children. She is active in the community and has her own radio show. She finds time for everyone else but is too busy to pay attention to her health.

"I'm always tired and don't have any energy," she told Dr. Whatling.

"It's no wonder," the doctor said lightheartedly. "You're running after your kids all day long, you have your radio show, and you make time for your husband."

"That's true, but these things give me energy," Kate said. "I also make it a priority to get eight hours of sleep each night. But this is a feeling of being weak."

"Do you have chest pain, shortness of breath, cough, or abdominal pain?"

"No," Kate said, "I don't have any other symptoms and I'm not depressed."

"Your blood pressure is normal, and your heart and lungs are normal," Dr. Whatling said. "Your weight is borderline increased and the extra amount seems to be belly weight. The increased abdominal weight is the risky type."

"I knew about the increased weight and was too busy to do anything about it."

"Do you do any type of exercise?"

"I don't have an exercise routine," Kate said. "The kids keep me running. The rest of the time, I'm in front of the computer working on my radio show."

"How are the kids?"

"My daughter's great, but my son, Craig, complains of being tired and sometimes has an upset stomach."

"Sounds like we have some work to do to find out what's going on with the two of you."

———

In the next chapters, each of the five vital steps will be discussed in detail as you learn how to manage your nutrition. You'll also learn more about Kate and her son, Craig.

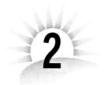

Good Nutrition Takes Know-How:
Read, Listen, and Learn

Learn everything you can about nutrition. Read books, listen to CDs in your car, search the internet, and monitor social media sites. New developments occur every day, and importantly, old myths are being updated, many proven wrong. This knowledge will give you a basis for a successful long-term nutrition program.

Let's begin with carbohydrate, fat, and protein metabolism. You'll also learn about fiber, vitamins, minerals, food hormones, anti-inflammatory foods, reading labels, and food safety.

We need good carbohydrates. We don't need the bad-quantity ones. They cause fat deposition and inflammation. About one-half of our diet is derived from carbohydrates. Their main purpose is to provide fuel for the body and brain, and they're fundamental for blood glucose sugar control. For successful nutrition management, you should know the good ones. And to avoid life-threatening diseases, you should learn about the bad-quantity carbs.

———

Brad complained to the nutritionist that he continued to gain weight even though he'd been eating nothing. The nutritionist didn't believe it until Brad explained the details. He wasn't eating anything solid, but he was drinking his food and in a surprisingly large amount—five huge 30- to 40-ounce containers of sodas and fruit "smoothies" every day.

A 32-ounce sugar cola may contain 310 calories, but one super-sized, 40-ounce fruit smoothie can have an astounding 1,500 calories! You do the math: Brad was drinking five sodas and smoothies—4,000 to 6,000 calories a day. It won't take long to pack on the pounds.

Furthermore, the amount of processed white sugar and saturated fats can be astronomical in sodas and smoothies, which can rapidly cause inflamed, clogged arteries and cardiovascular disease.

——

Carbohydrates include monosaccharides, which are the simple, one-molecule sugars such as glucose, fructose found in fruit, and galactose in milk. The disaccharides are two simple sugar molecules and include sucrose and lactose. Polysaccharides are long-chain simple sugars.

Sucrose is table sugar made up of glucose and fructose that are split by the sucrase enzyme in the small intestine. Lactose in milk is split into galactose and glucose by lactase. That's the enzyme that diminishes in adults and causes abdominal discomfort and other abdominal symptoms as milk and milk products are no longer easily digested.

——

Glucose is the simple sugar used for quick energy by the muscles, heart, and brain. It's the sugar that causes insulin release to keep the blood sugar glucose level in a healthy range. Glucose is metabolized in the small intestine and provides instant energy. Extra glucose is stored in the muscles and liver as glycogen polysaccharide, and is the equivalent of starch in plants.

One of the answers to weight gain is that extra glucose left over after quick energy use and glycogen formation is stored as fat. That's why eating extra portions of starchy foods and carbohydrates causes the fat around the middle. A person needs a balance of carbohydrate for fast energy and glycogen, but not the extra helpings and portions for fat production.

Before we go on from glucose metabolism, it would be helpful to learn about an insulin surge or insulin spike. What is it? Can it be harmful?

Insulin is a hormone produced by the pancreas beta cells and is released when the blood glucose is high. It transports glucose out of the blood into the cells to provide energy. Some carbohydrates such as white table sugar or sugary foods cause high spikes in the blood glucose level, causing an insulin surge to normalize the blood glucose level. If not burned up or stored as glycogen, this extra glucose turns to fat.

Insulin also stimulates synthesis of fat storage triglycerides from free fatty acids, and high blood triglyceride levels cause rigid arteries prone to inflammation and cardiovascular disease.

An insulin spike also can overshoot and cause too much glucose transport to the cells, leaving the blood glucose low, which can activate a cortisol response from the adrenal glands to stabilize the blood glucose level. A minor cortisol response may cause a transient burst of energy, but a chronic high cortisol response can lead to inflammation and weight gain.

Glucagon is a hormone secreted by the pancreas alpha cells and its action is opposite from insulin—it's secreted when the blood glucose is low. It raises the blood sugar level by releasing glucose from glycogen stored in the liver. When blood sugar is low, it may also signal fat cells to convert triglycerides into fatty acids.

It's important also to learn about the glycemic index. This is determined by measuring the blood glucose after giving a person a specific food and measuring the blood glucose level for a period of time afterward. A high glycemic index means the food causes a high glucose level, resulting in an insulin spike, while a low glycemic index means no increase in blood glucose after eating the food. Low glycemic food is a source of energy, while high glycemic food can cause fat storage and synthesis of triglycerides, causing inflamed arteries. Some high glycemic foods include baked goods, highly refined foods, white bread, mashed white potatoes, French fries, and white rice. Some of these foods can be prepared to have low glycemic indexes.

The dangerous insulin-surge effect of high-glycemic foods can be countered by eating them along with foods containing protein, healthy fats, and fiber that can slow absorption, preventing the insulin spike.

———

Fructose is the sweet sugary taste found in fruit. Its metabolic pathway differs from glucose because fructose is metabolized in the liver, and in healthy portions, doesn't cause the harmful insulin surge, cortisol release, and fat deposition.

However, there is no insulin regulation so too much high-fructose corn syrup can be as dangerous as table sugar. This is because the excess fructose is stored as triglycerides, which can lead to direct vascular injury, insulin-resistance, and type 2 diabetes. The manufacturing of this highly concentrated 55% fructose became popular in the 1960s. In small quantities, it may not be harmful, but it's everywhere and too much can increase your triglyceride level. It's in processed foods, soft drinks, pastries, cereals, breads, snacks, candy bars, energy bars, lunch meats, yogurts, and even soups. So, it's easy to eat or drink large amounts.

Another important thing to remember is that foods that are labeled "lite" do not necessarily mean fewer calories or healthier; the word means light in color.

Complex carbohydrates are 20 or more sugar units chained together. Enzymes attack one end so they take a long time to break down, and therefore do not cause the insulin surge response. Refined carbohydrates such as white flour and white rice no longer have the outer coat that contains healthy fiber and magnesium.

Fiber is a special carbohydrate that needs a separate review.

———

Phil had a cranky abdominal system. He experienced gassy bowel rumblings with cramps and constipation so bad that it caused bleeding hemorrhoids.

"Do I need surgery for these hemorrhoids?" Phil asked Dr. Lewis.

"Let's review your eating habits."

"What does that have to do with surgery?" Phil asked. "I eat typical meat and potatoes, and sometimes some fast-food hamburgers, French fries, and smoothies."

"Yes, that sounds like the typical diet," Dr. Lewis said. "What about fiber?"

"What's fiber? Rabbit food?"

"You're close," the doctor replied with a smile. "There's insoluble fiber in foods like wheat bran that will regulate the bowels, and soluble fiber in oatmeal that can lower your low-density lipoprotein or LDL-carrying cholesterol, which is the lipoprotein capable of causing vascular inflammation."

"Sounds like a lot of action for eating cardboard," Phil said as he visualized the health-food meals he had seen on TV.

They talked about foods that contain these fibers and how much was needed. Phil learned about reading food labels and searching for fiber content. The doctor told Phil to increase fiber slowly at first and drink water, because fiber can gum up the works if taken too much and too fast.

Phil returned for his six-week follow-up.

"I had trouble at first," he told the doctor, "but once I got used to it, it was a miracle. My abdominal noises and agony settled down with no cramps and the bowel evened out on a regular basis."

"That's what I like to hear," Dr. Lewis said. "Should we go ahead with that hemorrhoid surgery?"

"Not a chance," Phil said emphatically. "They're gone."

———

Although it may be like eating cardboard, fiber is powerful. The two types of fiber are special carbohydrates that have multiple benefits. Fiber can make you feel full. It can even out blood sugar levels and prevent the metabolic syndrome and prediabetes because it slows the absorption of sugar. And, the overall glycemic index is decreased, which prevents insulin surges.

Insoluble fiber is the woody portion of plant-based foods, such as broccoli and asparagus stems, and can regulate bowel function. These insoluble fibers can lower the risk of hemorrhoids, irritable bowel syndrome, and diverticulosis from less straining.

Soluble fiber is the gummy substance in oatmeal and red beans. It forms a gel with water, and beta-glucan in soluble fiber can decrease the blood level of low-density lipoprotein (LDL).

Fiber is important for people of all ages. The daily amount of total fiber is about 35 grams for men and 25 for women, and slightly less after age 50, with 30 grams for men and 20 for women. It's important to drink water when increasing the fiber content because it can develop a bezoar ball in the stomach of nondigestible substance, especially if a supplement such as psyllium is used too rapidly. Eat fruits and vegetables with the peel. Add lentils and beans. Use brown rice instead of white rice and have high-fiber breakfast cereals for breakfast.

———

It's time to learn about fats. Which of the fats are the good ones and which are the bad-quantity ones? What are the omega-3 fatty acids?

Fats, also called lipids, are energy-dense with nine calories per gram, while carbohydrates and protein have four calories per gram.

Healthy fats have many functions. They provide a huge source of energy; form cellular structures; protect internal organs such as the brain and heart; function in the skin as insulation; carry fat-soluble vitamins A, D, E, and K; and they are needed for production of regulatory hormones.

Fats are made up of a long string of a three-fatty acid glycerol backbone. Saturated fats mean the long chain is saturated with hydrogen ions so there is no space for other bonds. They are in the solid white form at room temperature like lard and the white fat on a steak, but some are liquid, like coconut oil and palm oil, that become solid when cold, as in ice cream. Other saturated fats are in cheese, pastries, and whole milk.

Saturated fats are the dangerous ones because they become low-density fatty-containing molecules referred to as lipoproteins in the blood that cause inflammation and plaques in the arteries. These plaques can occlude the artery or break off, causing artery occlusion elsewhere. If the artery supplies blood to the heart or brain, the tissue supplied by the artery receives no oxygen and dies, leading to heart attacks and strokes.

The unsaturated fats are the healthy ones, but pay attention, because one of them, trans fat, is not so healthy. Unsaturated fats have empty bonding sites in the long string of fatty acids. These empty sites can combine with oxygen, making the food rancid. That's what happens to olive oil if left out too long in the air. Monosaturated fats have one bond available and polyunsaturated fats have two or more available bonds. These healthy unsaturated fats are liquid at room temperature.

Omega-3 fatty acids are a group of several fatty acids classified as essential fatty acids because we need them. The name is derived from the location of the first double bond—three carbons in from the end. Omega-3 fatty acids are needed for prostaglandins, which are lipid-based substances with many healthy functions, and omega-3 fatty acids have an anti-inflammatory action. They reduce cardiovascular disease by maintaining elasticity and softness of blood vessels. Omega-3 fatty acids are found in cold-water fish and plant oils such as flaxseed.

Omega-6 fatty acids, just like the omega-3 fatty acids, are essential fatty acids. The name derivation is easy. The first double bond occurs at the sixth spot. In appropriate amounts, they are good for the heart and brain, but unlike omega-3 fatty acids, too much can cause inflammation and cardiovascular disease. It's the high omega-6-to-omega-3 ratio that is hazardous so it's important to keep a balance between these two fatty acid groups.

Beware of trans fats. They occur naturally in tiny amounts in some foods, but most are manufactured by adding hydrogen ions to the empty bonds in unsaturated fats so the food becomes more solid, like fully saturated fats. It's added to commercial foods so they don't become spoiled or rancid as quickly. Trans fat can be found in stick margarine and processed foods such as commercially baked cookies, muffins, pies, and cakes, and in fried foods such as doughnuts and french fries. These trans fats act just like saturated fats, leading to inflamed artery walls and plaques.

What are triglycerides? The body stores fatty acids as triglycerides, which can be measured in the blood and are sometimes referred to as your "trig" level.

Are triglycerides harmful? Yes, excessive levels in the blood are harmful and may be even more harmful as a cause of artery wall inflammation than the saturated fats.

High trig levels are caused by the body failing to burn up the food that's consumed because the leftover is stored as triglycerides. If you have a healthy weight and exercise, you burn up most of the calories from food, so the triglyceride storage is at a healthy level, available when needed.

If the calories are not burned up, the triglyceride level in the blood increases, which has a direct damaging way of injuring blood vessels by making them stiff and inflamed—prone to being clogged up, causing heart attacks and strokes.

You'll be surprised, but it's not fatty food intake that can cause an increase in the blood triglyceride level. It's the bad-quantity carbs. Foods that cause high trig levels include processed and sugary foods, like baked goods, and foods made from white flour, such as pasta, breads, and crackers.

———

Protein is the third big metabolic food that you need to learn about. It's mostly good, but you need to keep track of the company it keeps.

Protein is made up of amino acids and is reduced to its individual amino acids during the digestive process. There are about 10,000 proteins in the body, and they are essential for every tissue in the body, in the skin, hair, bone, and muscles. Proteins contain nitrogen, so the waste product is urea in the urine

Your genes contain instructions to produce these proteins from among 20 amino acids. There are essential amino acids that the body cannot make, such as lysine and tryptophan, and the nonessential amino acids that the body can make, such as aspartic acid, glutamine, glycine, and tyrosine.

Proteins have numerous functions, such as building and repairing tissue; acting as structural elements as collagen in the skin and actin and myocin in muscle; providing immune function; synthesizing hundreds of enzymes; and helping to build hormones.

Proteins are also blood transporters. Albumin transports drugs, vitamins, and minerals. If blood albumin is low, drug levels can be increased, causing an adverse reaction. Low albumin can result in water leaking into the cells, causing edema, swelling of the ankles, and even the abdomen. The blood protein, transferrin, is an iron transporter. Proteins also carry fat in the blood, and these are called the lipoproteins.

Protein is a secondary source of energy after carbohydrates are depleted. The nitrogen is stripped off in the liver and the protein is turned into carbohydrate.

Protein can't be stored, so we need daily intake. If the intake is insufficient, muscle and immune system function can be lost.

Some foods, such as chicken and fish, have complete protein, which means these foods contain all 20 amino acids. Some vegetables, such as quinoa and soy bean, have complete protein. Incomplete proteins, such as found in bread, lack one or more amino acids, and additional protein is needed. If one amino acid is missing, protein synthesis will stop; therefore, a balance of protein foods is needed to provide all 20 amino acids.

Protein deficiency disorders include anorexia nervosa and kwashiorkor or marasmus in the very severe malnourished form. These disorders are characterized by low albumin levels in the blood, which result in muscle wasting and a poor immune system prone to serious infections.

———

You need to know about vitamins not only because you need to have the right amount of the right types, but also because you can take too much of some of them. There are two types. The water-soluble vitamins are the B complex and C, and the fat-soluble vitamins are A, D, E, and K.

The B vitamins have all types of function. There are eight of them and they function as coenzymes, providing catalysts to metabolized foods to produce energy. Thiamin is B_1 and helps with glucose and protein metabolism and in synthesis of the neurotransmitters, which are the chemicals used to transmit nerve impulses within the brain and to the muscles. An old disease called beriberi can occur if a person is deficient in this vitamin.

Riboflavin is B_2, which is involved in carbohydrate, protein, and fat metabolism. Niacin is B_3 and is a coenzyme in many metabolic reactions.

Pyridoxine, or vitamin B_6, is a coenzyme, especially for protein synthesis and neurotransmitters development. Excessive supplemental amounts of B_6 can be toxic.

———

Brenda was a competitive tennis player who took a large amount of vitamin B_6 supplement because she had heard it would help to improve her speed and accuracy. But the unexpected happened. She lost her tennis-racket grip from neurotransmitter muscle weakness. Fortunately, the vitamin B_6 toxicity was discovered early, before permanent damage had occurred. There's plenty of vitamin B_6 in foods such as spinach and other vegetables.

———

Vitamin B_{12} is stored in the liver, so only a small amount is needed, and conversely it takes years to develop a vitamin B_{12} deficiency. This vitamin has the important function of maintaining healthy hemoglobin in the blood and stabilizing the central nervous system. B_{12} deficiency will cause a large, fragile red blood cell anemia and neurological dysfunction. As this vitamin needs an intrinsic factor produced in the stomach, individuals who have gastric bypass surgery will need a supplemental source.

Folic acid is also a B vitamin, and deficiency causes a type of anemia like B_{12}, characterized by large, fragile red blood cells. An important function of folic acid is its ability to maintain a safe blood level of homocysteine, which is an amino acid created by metabolism. For cardiovascular health, healthy folic acid intake prevents high blood levels of homocysteine that can cause inflamed arteries, leading to cardiovascular diseases and heart attacks. Healthy amounts of B_6 and B_{12} also help maintain a healthy homocysteine level.

Vitamin C is ascorbic acid and the other water-soluble vitamin. It's an antioxidant and reduces the amount of reactive compounds in the body, helping to prevent cardiovascular disease and inflammatory disease. Vitamin C helps with collagen synthesis used in scar-tissue formation, blood vessels, and cartilage; and it's involved in creating neurotransmitters. It donates electrons during reactions and can keep iron and copper atoms in their healthy reduced states. Vitamin C can contribute to a healthy functioning immune system, and even has anti-histamine effects.

Among the fat-soluble vitamins, Vitamin A has traditionally been good for the eyes and vision, but you can take too much. The skin can turn yellow-orange, and if the excess is severe, blurred vision may develop.

Vitamin D acts like a hormone and is a key component of bone health. Deficiency can cause rickets, but too much supplemental vitamin D can be toxic.

Vitamin E is primarily an antioxidant vitamin that can be obtained with healthy diet sources. Vitamin K is used for the normal coagulation of the blood.

———

Minerals are essential to good nutrition. You need sodium, potassium, calcium, magnesium, iron, zinc, and selenium, and a healthy diet with vegetables can supply them.

Too much sodium is the most dangerous hazard for people these days. Yes, the body needs a small amount, but sodium is everywhere. It's obviously in table salt, but it's also in processed foods, cheeses, cured and smoked meats, and in juice drinks. A small can of spicy tomato juice can have 1,500 milligrams of salt. That's all you need for the entire day, and it's in an 8-ounce drink. Read the labels. Look for sodium and keep it as low as possible.

Potassium is needed for the body's electrical system, especially for maintenance of a healthy heart rhythm. Potassium can also help manage excessive sodium intake because an equal amount of potassium will neutralize the same amount of sodium. Potassium is the mineral in bananas and other fruits and vegetables. Too low and too high blood values can be dangerous, as they will cause serious heart arrhythmias. A healthy diet that includes fruits and vegetables usually includes sufficient potassium. Diuretic medications can decrease potassium, sometimes dangerously low, while other medications can increase it.

Calcium is needed for healthy bones, especially in connection with vitamin D, and the prevention of osteoporosis.

Magnesium is an amazing element, often underestimated, and functions as a muscle relaxant. It blocks too much calcium from entering nerve cells, keeping them in a non-excited state. That's why milk of magnesia relieves constipation; it relaxes the muscles surrounding the colon. And that's why muscle spasms and cramps can occur with a magnesium deficiency. Like vitamins, magnesium participates in many enzyme actions involving carbohydrate, fat, and protein metabolism. Importantly, healthy levels of magnesium can keep the arteries soft and pliable, countering the stiff and hardening effects from too much triglyceride and low-density lipoproteins in the blood.

Manganese is similar to magnesium and just as important. It's involved as a coenzyme in building healthy bone structure and may have an anti-inflammatory action. It helps in carbohydrate, fat, and protein metabolism. Manganese is found in whole grains, vegetables, and the legumes such as beans and peas.

Iron is the basic molecule forming hemoglobin and hemoglobin is key for carrying oxygen in your blood. It's found in vegetables such as spinach.

Zinc is needed for a healthy immune system and is involved in wound healing. It's found in whole grain foods.

Selenium, an obscure mineral, is needed in small amounts and functions in the development of antioxidant enzymes. It's found in vegetables and the amount varies according to where the vegetables were grown and the amounts of selenium in the soil.

Iodine has become a forgotten essential element. It was added to table salt as a public health measure during the 20th century for the prevention of goiter, and that's the problem. Table salt can quickly add to your daily sodium intake. The higher the sodium intake, the higher the rate of heart attacks and strokes. We only need a tiny amount of iodine, 150 micrograms, but we need it daily because iodine is not stored. People who eat healthy foods will consume the perfect amount. Supplements are not needed, especially because this element can be consumed at too high a level. Iodine is common in soil, and iodine deficiency occurs in countries and locations with no iodine in the soil. Most foods have some iodine. Foods that contain higher amounts include ocean fish, seaweed from salad or wrapped in sushi, asparagus, carrots, tomatoes, peas, cabbage, spinach, squash, beans, bananas, and strawberries.

——

Next, we'll explore the effects of appetite hormones.

Ghrelin is the hunger hormone released from the stomach lining and pancreas that signals the brain to eat more. High-calorie, processed foods increase ghrelin release, which prompts us to eat more of these foods. Stress also causes increased ghrelin release. Additionally, lack of sleep can cause an increase in ghrelin and can lead to an elevated appetite and weight gain.

Leptin is the appetite suppressor hormone made in the adipocytes, or fat cells, and signals your brain's hypothalamus to stop eating. If individuals are born without the leptin-producing gene, they are prone to extreme obesity. And individuals who are extremely overweight have high levels of leptin because the overstuffed fat cells become resistant to the appetite-suppressing effects. Also, highly concentrated fructose corn syrups may impede the appetite-suppressing effects of leptin. Lack of sleep appears to decrease the leptin level.

Adiponectin is an obscure regulatory hormone in the body, and its function may surprise you—it burns up glucose. Adiponectin is produced in the adipocytes and regulates lipid and glucose metabolism, so it speeds up metabolism, burning glucose instead of producing fat storage. It has an anti-inflammatory response, which is phenomenal because it can protect the interior walls of arteries, preventing coronary artery disease.

Healthy, normal-size fat cells produce adequate amounts of this hormone. But, if these fat cells are stuffed to overflowing capacity, problems can develop. First, low levels of adiponectin will result in insulin resistance and diabetes, and loss of its anti-inflammatory action can cause inflamed arteries and cardiovascular disease. Second, if the fat cells become too filled up, their membrane may not function appropriately, triggering direct inflammatory effects. Third, as you may remember from the leptin comments, overstuffed fat cells limit leptin's function of suppressing the appetite. Maintain a healthy weight for well-functioning fat-storage cells.

———

Alex ate lean protein foods and foods containing omega-3 fatty acids and fiber, and he had strong, soft, flexible blood vessels that will last for a very long time.

Andrew ate processed foods, fried foods, and foods filled with saturated fats, and he had calcified rocks in his blood vessels, setting him up for a potential heart attack.

Alex ate foods that did not cause inflammation and that blocked toxic effects of foods that cause inflammation. Andrew ate foods that can cause inflammation.

———

Can what you eat make such a huge difference? Yes, and way beyond what you can imagine. You know about the foods that cause inflammation—high-saturated fat foods, trans fat, processed foods, and sugar-laden foods.

So, let's examine the anti-inflammatory foods.

Flavonoids are the color foods, and make up a group of naturally occurring compounds found in colorful yellow, red, and purple fruits, and vegetables such as spinach and kidney beans. They can keep your blood vessels flexible by inhibiting synthesis of the low-density fatty lipoproteins. Citrin can, too. It's sometimes referred to as "Vitamin P", and is the most active flavonoid in the citrus fruit, the lemon.

Herbs and spices. Are they healthy, neutral or harmful? Most are neutral, although some, such as turmeric in curry powder and ginger, may have anti-inflammatory action and prevent arterial plaque formation. Some, such as rosemary, may act as antioxidants and prevent formation of the toxic compounds produced in grilled, broiled, or fried foods.

———

Is it possible that if Eva ate certain foods and avoided certain types of foods, she could prevent cancer? The answer is probably yes and confirmation of that is emerging. You can surmise the foods that could increase the risk of cancer: They're the grilled, charred, or cured meats that create toxic nitrosamines, and the high-saturated-fat foods, such as processed meats and trans fat-containing foods.

Aflatoxin from foods contaminated with *Aspergillus* molds, such as peanuts and whole grains, is a cause of liver cancer. This is an extremely rare possibility, but it shows the importance of clean food production and not producing foods such as grains or grapes that have developed fungal or mold growth.

Those are the bad ones for potentially causing cancer. What about the good ones? They're the right types of fatty acids, with omega-3 fatty acids on top of the list. Surprisingly, increased fiber intake can decrease colon and rectal cancer risk, not because the fiber itself is an anticancer agent, but because regular soft stools don't allow toxic waste products from foods or produced by bacteria to remain in the colon long enough to cause inflammation or cell mutations. Fiber moves everything through the intestines faster. Fiber also binds to toxic cancer-producing substances and neutralizes them.

Eating whole grains appears to decrease the risk of prostate cancer, while refined-grain foods have no effect. Think brightly colored fruits and vegetables—the bright yellows, oranges, reds, green, blues, and purples—they can potentially decrease cancer risk. Soy and soy-based products can contain anti-cancer ingredients.

Next, we'll examine probiotics and prebiotics. You might be surprised to learn that probiotics are bacteria—millions of them. They're the good bacteria that are necessary for healthy digestion. A healthy diet that includes vegetables is usually sufficient to restore and maintain the good bacteria needed for digestion. Fermented foods such as yogurt, sauerkraut, kimchi, and tempeh are sources of probiotics, but it's important to read the label, as yogurt may contain high amounts of sugar and high-fructose corn syrup, and excessive sodium may be found in foods such as kimchi and sauerkraut.

Prebiotics are even more surprising. They're foods that feed these bacteria, and include fiber found in artichokes and asparagus.

A relatively new development in nutrition is the oxygen radical absorbance capacity, or ORAC, score, which is designed to measure the antioxidant level of a food. High scores mean foods are high in antioxidants that can neutralize oxygen free radicals, which can cause inflammation of blood vessels, joints, and other organ systems of the body. Blueberries and strawberries top the list of fruits with high scores, while kale and spinach top the list of vegetables.

It's helpful to review the meaning of organic foods. They may be good for you. This is not just a trendy term, but it means that foods are grown by specific methods established by the U.S. Department of Agriculture, or USDA. Look for the green label on organic foods. Read labels carefully; the term "all natural" does not mean organic.

The 1990 Farm Bill established the standards for producing and handling foods labeled as organic. Organic meat, poultry, eggs, and dairy products are derived from animals that are given no antibiotics or growth hormones.

Rotational grazing and mixed-forage pastures are used for livestock. Organic foods are produced without pesticides or fertilizers that are made with synthetic ingredients. Crop rotations are used to fertilize the soil. A government-approved inspector must certify the farm or ranch. An inspector must also certify companies that handle and process the foods.

Next, we'll examine food labels.

It takes time at first, but you can develop a phenomenal nutritional program by reading labels. Once you know them, you won't have to reread them, so the process will become easier and quicker.

There are three factors when reading food labels. First, what is the portion size? Some single-serving pizzas have a one-quarter slice as the portion size, but you usually assume the percentage elements are for the whole pizza. It doesn't make sense, but some standard-size candy bar may contain five to seven portions. Check the portion size. Also, remember that the front of the box or package is usually advertising. It's not the official label. All natural does not mean organic.

Second, read the nutrient list with an eye toward saturated fats, sodium, sugar, and fiber content.

Third, read the ingredient list at the bottom of the label and look for high-fructose corn syrup, sugar alcohols, saturated fatty oils, and for specific allergens such as nuts.

A good food label will tell you that the food contains—per serving—fewer than 300 calories and five grams of fat and no saturated fat, no trans fat, carbohydrates of fewer than 25 grams, sugar of fewer than 8 grams, sodium of fewer than 200 milligrams, protein of more than 10 grams, and fiber of more than 3 grams.

What's BPA? Is it harmful? BPA is bisphenol A. It's an organic chemical used to make plastics and epoxy resins for consumer products such as food and beverage containers. It's been called an endocrine-disrupting chemical. BPA may leach from the epoxy resins lining cans of liquid baby formula and canned foods such as soups or pasta. Hard plastic food and drink containers may contain BPA. Some metal water bottles may be lined with BPA-containing plastics. Continue your awareness of this issue.

Food safety can be learned quickly. Learn the basic rules.

Topping the list is washing hands with soap–preferably for about 20 seconds, that is, long enough to sing the alphabet song.

Don't leave foods out too long. *Staphylococcus* toxic food poisoning can develop easily in creamy casseroles, chowders, or chicken or tuna salad sandwiches left at room temperature or for outside eating. There are three basic time periods. Less than two hours at room temperature, less than one hour at 90 degrees, and only a few minutes at 130 degrees, which can readily occur in your vehicle's trunk on a hot day. If you're in doubt, throw it out.

You've now learned some facts about food that can be helpful in managing your nutrition. Before we address the subject of the diagnostic process, we'll explain the "belly brain."

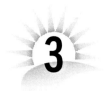

Your "Belly Brain" Is Trying to Tell You Something

Everyone has a belly brain. It's very much like a second brain. It's called the enteric nervous system—the separate but interconnected nervous system that works along your entire intestinal tract, your mouth, and to a lesser extent, your gallbladder and pancreas. There are as many neurons in your enteric nervous system as in your spinal cord, which gives the system the ability to convey a ton of information.

That's why, to manage your nutrition, you should learn how it works.

Science has known about the enteric nervous system for more than 100 years, but most of us still perceive the brain in our heads as being in control of our bodies. In fact, more information passes from your belly brain to your head brain than vice versa. If you're surprised by that, consider such established adages in Western culture as having a gut feeling about something or someone. In many Eastern cultures also, people will tap their stomachs when they're asked where they think.

Let's listen to our belly brain for a minute.

Think in your mind about eating a greasy food. How does your stomach react? Now think about a banana. How does your stomach react?

That's the belly brain talking to you. It may not speak English or in full sentences, but it's definitely giving you an opinion. That's a distressed "no" for the greasy food and a calming "yes" for the banana.

Why does the belly brain have to be so powerful? The gut has to assess everything we take into our bodies and figure out what to do with it. What part of what we've eaten is vitamins? What part is made up of other nutrients? What part is fuel? How much insulin does the pancreas need to make? How much bile is needed from the gallbladder? Should our body use what's come in immediately, or should it be stored for a time when it would be better to digest? Is something we've taken in a threat or a toxin?

These seem like straightforward issues to address, but they're complex. Nutritionists acknowledge that they don't know yet how everything works together, but a few dynamics between what we take in and how our bodies use it have become clear.

One important dynamic is the interplay between stress and digestion. Insulin, a hormone made by the pancreas, works to push sugar into cells from the blood stream. When we're relaxed and our calming parasympathetic nervous system pathways dominate, we make the right amount of insulin to digest what we eat. But when we're stressed, our hyped-up sympathetic nervous system takes over, and cortisol is the hormone activated. We not only signal our digestion to move more slowly or come to a halt, we make more insulin and the cortisol level goes up. Unknowingly, when the body feels high stress constantly, these two hormones work together to store fat and add weight. And that high cortisol causes inflammation.

High cortisol levels influence the cephalic, or head phase, of digestion, which accounts for about 40% to 60% of total digestion. The cephalic phase includes sensory details gleaned from taste, aroma, visual appreciation of food, and our pleasure with it. When we're looking forward to a meal and smelling it as it cooks, our mouths water in anticipation, readying our bodies to take in all those nutrients.

For some people, anticipation of a meal is such a powerful thing that they start producing insulin just thinking about it, which is called the cephalic phase insulin response. But when we're stressed and the excitable sympathetic nervous system dominates, cortisol desensitizes our bodies to pleasure, whether from touch or taste. As we decrease our ability to taste or anticipate and experience pleasure from a meal, we inhibit our ability to get the nutrients we need from our food. Eventually, we're going to need to eat more, which means our bodies need to produce more insulin. All those extra calories consumed cause insulin surges that not only cause weight gain but can lead to cellular inflammation.

Our emotions and certain psychological archetypes also influence how we approach eating, our cephalic phase, and can cause stress. Sometimes we are children who eat for comfort. Sometimes we eat to act as victims, thinking that we might as well overeat because no one will love us whether we're thin or heavy. Sometimes you might play the rebel and say, "I'll eat what I want, and who are you to tell me differently?" Sometimes we are wolves who devour our food. And sometimes we're cold scientists, who regard food as fuel and nothing else.

Unfortunately though, the fat that is deposited from eating under stress usually goes right to the middle. We can feel increased bloating, indigestion, and damaging gastrointestinal reflux.

But before you think you're in thrall to your belly brain, remember that your head brain can influence the system, too.

If stress deprives you of nutrients and causes weight gain, and all the problems that go with that, you can take concrete steps to give better signals to your belly brain. Ask yourself if you're about to eat while stressed. If the answer is yes, try to figure out why. Start with: Who's eating? The rebel? The child? Pretend instead that you're a healthy, strong person who eats in a dignified, self-respecting manner.

In addition to this sort of visualization, try to take three to five belly breaths to fool your belly brain into thinking you're calm. A belly breath moves your lower abdomen outward with each deep breath. Or play some music. Focus one of your senses on something calming, like candles, palm trees, or a soft sand beach.

You should try an ancient yogic technique, which is to eat only until you've reached thermic efficiency. This means to eat until your body has taken in enough fuel to satisfy your energy needs, which is a feeling you can train your mind to sense, just before you start to feel really heavy and full. This is a fantastic concept. Eat to your high-energy level, not to your over-full level.

Above all, slow down while you eat. Your body considers food that's consumed too fast a stressor all by itself. You might have heard of the French paradox. That even though the French diet consists of more fat per person per year than Americans and other cultures, the French on average show lower rates of diabetes, obesity, and cardiovascular disease.

Researchers found it was the red wine—and there is benefit to the colors red and purple in foods such as grapes, cranberries, and blueber-ries. But nutritionists believe that French people generally take pleasure in their food. They tend to eat longer and more relaxed meals at midday, which is a time when the body is programmed to digest and extract all the nutrients from food most efficiently. In fact, you can optimize weight loss and calorie-burning by taking advantage of this natural body rhythm and eating the majority of your calories in the first half of the day.

A large breakfast is especially useful because the belly brain reacts by digesting the food efficiently, smoothing out the insulin surges and not storing fat. If you're eating at 10 at night, you're not burning calories efficiently, which can result in fat deposition, and you're not giving your digestive system the nightly time of repair and rejuvenation.

Our bodies also fall into other natural rhythms. For example, we have a rhythm that revolves around the seasons. Most people naturally start shedding pounds in the spring and then start putting on weight in the fall in preparation for winter. Before our modern age in which we have central heating, summer and fall meant the time to gather fruits and vegetables, and it was time to store fat for the winter. Knowing this natural occurrence can reduce the stress about seasonal weight changes and the negative spiral of eating incorrectly.

Another natural rhythm involves growth and maintenance, which applies to adults as well as growing children. If you exercise or lift weights, your body goes into a building phase, and you feel more vigorous and put on muscle. The times in between are for maintenance, during which your body stays relatively the same. There are also seasonal changes as there is a subtle building phase during the spring.

So how we eat our food and when we eat our food can be as important as what we eat. Is your eating schedule healthy or does it lead to overeating the wrong foods? Modern life has led to a wealth of choices in supermarkets, but many of these choices do not involve high-quality foods.

Poor-quality foods contain refined and processed carbohydrates such as sugar, sugary cereals and pastries, snack foods, candy, and soft drinks. And there are poor-quality foods that contain high levels of saturated fats and trans fat, such as processed meats, bacon, pepperoni, potato chips, and french fries. Foods cooked at extremely high temperatures are an associated group of poor-quality foods.

Our digestive system is not equipped to handle these foods efficiently. They count only as calories devoid of healthy nutrients. And worse, these inefficient processes generate cellular inflammation and deposit fat throughout the body.

Foods cooked at extremely high temperatures that are fried, barbecued, or broiled can result in foods containing glycation end products. This glycation process occurs when glucose and proteins in foods are fused together and produce aberrant end products. These substances are not recognized naturally by our digestive system and can't be metabolized efficiently. The higher the saturated fat content in these foods, the higher the glycation rate is going to be from high-temperature cooking.

Glycation end products are in some packaged foods such as preheated products or frozen precooked meals.

These poorly metabolized substances, sometimes termed glycotoxins, can cause cellular inflammation throughout the body organs and especially the internal walls of the blood vessels, which can result in cardiovascular disease.

Diabetics are especially vulnerable to these effects. Diabetics who can maintain low levels of glycation end products often do not develop heart, kidney, or eye complications, while those with high levels may develop these complications. Yet a small percentage of diabetics with high levels of these glycation end products do not develop complications. This may mean that some glycation end products are not toxic. Or, interestingly, an individual may have the genetic-enabling enzyme to safely neutralize glycation end products. This latter explanation is a distinct possibility because we know that some individuals who lack one or more genes to produce a specific food enzyme can't metabolize that food. So the opposite can be true. Individuals may have one or more genes to produce enzymes to metabolize and neutralize toxic substances.

Steamed and slow, low-heat cooking can minimize these glycation substances, and certain vitamins and other substances found in vegetables and other foods can neutralize these glycation end products. As noted above, some individuals may genetically have the metabolic enzymes to detoxify these substances.

Milk products, eggs, and meats produced with the use of growth hormones and supplements also represent poor-quality foods, although in a different way. They might be packed with nutrients but they carry substances that can put our systems out of balance. Most animals raised for food are fed growth hormones to speed their time from birth to marketability and antibiotics to keep them healthy. Some may not be harmful to us. Yet whatever is fed to the cow who makes the milk, the hen who lays the eggs, or the animal or fish that becomes food is passed on to us. For example, the effect of animal growth hormones for us is weight gain.

Artificial sweeteners do not qualify as high-quality foods. For one thing, they have no nutritional value. They provide sweet taste and nothing else, and no studies have shown that they help people lose weight. Worse, people may consume excessive amounts of foods that contain these artificial sweeteners such as diet sodas, resulting in gum disease and tooth decay from the acidic carbonation.

The sweet taste in some artificial sweeteners activates the sweet-taste buds in the tongue that could result in an insulin surge. That surge may cause hypoglycemia because there is no new source of glucose, so this extra insulin triggers cortisol release, inflammation, and fat storage.

Nina learned about this. She had two big diet sodas for breakfast every day and wondered why she was dizzy, irritable, and cranky an hour or so later. Her blood sugar had plummeted to 60, when it should be around 100. Also, an insulin increase could occur in an individual with already high insulin levels from insulin resistance, so this new insulin release results in the fat-storage response, especially in overweight individuals.

Let's look at high-quality foods. First, they are simple, nonprocessed foods and foods without barcodes. They're grown as naturally as possible with personal attention. They're fruits and vegetables grown organically from well-cultivated fields without pesticides. They're from free-range chickens and cattle. They're free-swimming fish in rivers, lakes, and oceans. They're nonprocessed carbohydrates that have not been fructose-condensed by a manufacturing process, and oils that have not been hydrogenated.

The method for consuming high-quality foods is simpler than you'd think. Eat as close to nature and naturally produced food as you can.

Although it might seem strange to think of skin-care products as nutritional, you should be aware that anything you put on your skin will end up in your body. Again, use a product that is as close to nature as possible. Exercise and sweating can help detoxify the body, but once a substance is within you, it could take time to eliminate it. Take a steam; you can feel the toxins sweat away.

You can manage your nutrition. Listen to your belly brain. You've used your head brain to learn about nutrition in the first two chapters.

Before you learn about taking a nutrition inventory and the diagnostic approach to nutrition in the next chapter, let's talk about food intolerance and food allergies. There are important distinctions.

Food intolerance is an adverse reaction from a food that occurs each time the food is consumed, especially in high quantities. The immune system is not activated, so it's not a food allergy; and not everyone develops symptoms, so it's not food poisoning.

Genetics and differences in traditions among people in various cultures are the causes of food intolerances. There may be lack of a metabolic enzyme or chemical for the specific food from a disease or from lacking a gene sequence. For example, lactase deficiency leads to milk and dairy product intolerances. The lactase gene is lacking in up to 15% of Europeans and in 70% to 90% of Asians—explaining the high rates of dairy product intolerance.

———

Metabolic enzymes are essential.

Foster and his friends were talking about their upcoming weekend trip at their favorite college hangout in Los Angeles. Suddenly, Foster started talking nonsense, ran to his car, and drove away, completely out of control. He drove through city streets at dangerous speeds, ignoring all the rules, until he was finally forced to stop by the LA police. He spent the night in jail and recalled nothing of the night except seeing his friends and drinking one beer. This is an extreme but possible result of alcohol intolerance, as Foster lacked the gene to produce the enzyme, alcohol dehydrogenase.

———

Alcohol dehydrogenase deficiency causes intolerance to drinking alcohol, even a very small amount. The rate of this deficiency varies among people throughout the world and may be as high as 50% in some cultures. Friends and family can easily recognize this problem, but it's often too late. Fatal accidents could occur. Fortunately, people can now purchase a simple DNA test to determine if they lack or are deficient in the alcohol dehydrogenase gene sequence.

Food allergies can play an important role in nutrition management. The immune system misidentifies a food as harmful and produces an immune globulin, called an IgE antibody, to neutralize the food or allergen, which is often a protein. Each time this food is encountered, the IgE antibodies cause cells to release histamine and inflammatory chemicals, which in turn cause itchy eyes, runny nose, hives, and in extreme situations, breathing distress and anaphylactic shock.

The types of foods differ somewhat among children and adults. Children may be allergic to one or both milk proteins, casein or whey, or eggs, peanuts, tree nuts, and soybeans, while adults may be allergic to shellfish, tree nuts, fish, peanuts, and eggs. In a small group of highly allergic people, even a tiny amount of the food such as a peanut can cause a reaction, while in less sensitive people, small amounts of the food can be tolerated. Children may outgrow their allergies to milk or soy while adults usually do not lose their allergies. Retesting can be performed if loss of an allergy is suspected.

There is a rare but strange allergy referred to as exercise-induced food allergy. A person has a specific food such as a milkshake, then exercises, and soon begins to have itching and sometimes wheezing and hives. The management is not to eat two hours before exercising.

Food allergy symptoms are variable and include the well-known hives, but they can also be sinus congestion, postnasal drip, wheezing, upset stomach, and even depression.

It's important to correctly diagnose a food allergy because under-diagnosis can lead to unnecessary suffering and serious complications, and over-diagnosis or misdiagnosis can lead to wrong treatment and unnecessary medications.

Under-diagnosis occurs when appropriate testing is not obtained. A helpful part of diagnostic testing is for people to keep a food diary and record reactions. The skin-scratch test with a diluted amount of the suspected food has been the traditional approach. This test is very sensitive, which means it will detect a food allergy if you have one, which is good, but the test is not specific, which means the test may be positive but not from a true food allergy. As a result of this low specificity, the combination of a positive skin test and a corresponding food diary is used to confirm a true food allergy.

Skin testing generally is not performed for individuals who have developed anaphylaxis or acute respiratory failure to a food, and it's not performed for individuals with widespread eczema. Blood tests for food-specific IgE antibodies are available, and even these need to be correlated with the food reaction log.

In unusual situations, double-blind food challenge tests can be performed using an opaque capsule of the suspected food and other foods.

There are excellent testing guidelines that will lead to an accurate diagnosis of a food allergy. It may seem that a person can have an allergy to many foods, but in reality, most individuals are truly allergic to only one or two foods. Over-diagnosis can lead people to develop nutritional problems because false-positive skin testing has led them to avoid many nutrition-packed foods.

Another important reason for an accurate diagnosis is that there are several food allergy mimics. These include ingestion of excessive histamine and food additives such as monosodium glutamate, or MSG. The symptoms may be similar but these are not immune dysfunction reactions. Sulfites added to foods can cause an acute asthma attack in an asthmatic, not from an allergy to sulfites, but from the irritant sulfur dioxide that is produced from sulfite metabolism.

Now that you've learned a variety of details about nutrition, it's time to move on to the diagnostic process.

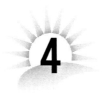

A Nutrition Inventory—Height, Weight, Body Fat—Leads to Diagnosis

At the beginning of the diagnostic process, it's important to take a nutrition inventory.

Begin with numbers. What's your height and weight? Find your healthy weight. Check the internet for tables, or use Dr. Hamwi's equation – for women, begin with 100 pounds for the first 5 feet and add 5 pounds for each inch over 5 feet. For men, begin with 106 pounds for the first 5 feet and add 6 pounds for each inch over 5 feet.

Calculate your body mass index, or BMI, which is a relationship between height and weight and works most of the time, although it may be misleading in muscular individuals or athletes. Enter your height and weight on an internet equation. A normal BMI is from 18.5 to 25; greater than 25 is overweight, 30 or greater is obese, and 40 or over is extreme obesity, while less than 18.5 is underweight.

Measure your waist circumference at your navel. Extra abdominal weight can be a risk factor for the metabolic syndrome, diabetes, heart disease, and stroke. Greater than 35 inches for women and greater than 40 inches for men is too much.

Measure your percentage of body fat. The body pod is an accurate method, although it may not be readily available. There are several alternatives, including body circumference measurements and skin-fold methods. One example is to use waist size at its narrowest point, waist size at the navel, hip size at its widest point, neck size, height, and weight. Programs on the internet can make the calculation for you. The body fat proportion should be less than 25% for women and less than 18% for men. High levels mean increased risk of diabetes and cardiovascular disease, especially if more than 35% for women and more than 25% for men.

Calculate your expected caloric intake. Take your ideal body weight and multiply it by ten to get your estimated basal metabolic rate, or BMR. Add up to 30% more calories if you are sedentary, 50% if moderately active, and 100% if active. You can use internet programs for accurate calculations.

Calculate the number of calories you burn up every day. The formula includes age, height, weight, and whether you are sedentary or active. It's simple. You don't want to eat more calories than you burn. Exercise will burn up calories, although not as much as you think; it's usually only 300 calories for an hour of exercise, and a snack can easily contain more than 300 calories. That's why exercise by itself will not result in weight loss, but it has many wonderful benefits, and it'll help maintain a healthy weight.

Most men burn 2,000 to 2,500 calories a day and most women burn 1,500 to 1,900 calories a day.

Determine the necessary calories for you and your calories burned. Do the math. It needs to be zero or you'll gain weight.

———

Let's learn about diagnosing the numerous nutrition-related diseases and disorders.

Three components of the diagnostic process include answering a series of questions, undergoing a physical examination, and diagnostic testing.

The major underweight conditions include protein malnutrition, or Kwashiorkor in its extreme, anorexia nervosa, and bulimia nervosa.

Anorexia develops in people who become obsessed with being thin. They may starve themselves or exercise excessively. For these individuals, thinness is equated with self-worth. Adolescent females are at the highest risk. Actors, dancers, models, and athletes such as runners, figure skaters, and gymnasts are also at high risk. The diagnosis is established by the questioning portion of the diagnostic process, as there is no single test. Criteria include refusal to maintain a healthy body weight, intense fear of gaining weight, and distorted body image.

Bulimia is an eating disorder in which a person binges on food and uses vomiting to prevent weight gain. This disorder has symptoms and risk factors similar to anorexia. Some people may have the two disorders simultaneously. Physical findings of dental cavities and gingivitis may be seen in individuals with bulimia because of the excessive exposure to stomach acid. There may be small cuts or calluses across the tops of the fingers from self-induced vomiting. The diagnostic criteria include binge eating and counteracting the binge eating with vomiting or medications with a frequency of at least twice a week for three months or more.

The major overweight-related disorders include metabolic syndrome, diabetes, coronary and peripheral vascular disease, and hypertension, along with their accompanying complications that include angina, heart attack, congestive heart failure, hypertensive heart disease, stroke, diabetic eye disease, and kidney failure.

Additional overweight disorders include arthritis of the hips and knees; gastroesophageal reflux disease, or GERD; gallbladder disease; polycystic ovary syndrome; obstructive sleep apnea, or OSA, which is frequent periods of not breathing at night; and increased risk for some types of cancers, such as colon cancer.

Metabolic syndrome is one of the fastest-growing, obesity-related health issues. It's defined as a combination of obesity, hypertension, abnormal blood lipid levels, and high blood sugar.

There are specific disorders of vitamin or mineral deficiencies as well as vitamin or mineral excess from taking too many supplements.

After meeting with your physician, you'll be asked a series of questions about your lifestyle, your family illnesses, your past illnesses, environmental questions, and questions about each organ system.

Did you ever smoke? For smokers, when did you start? How many packs per day did you smoke? When did you stop? Do you use alcohol? How much and how frequently? Are there any family members with any illnesses, and specifically, nutrition-related illnesses? Do you have any food intolerances? Do you have any food allergies? What are they and what happens?

What are the names and dosages of the medications, vitamins, or supplements that you take? When did you begin taking them?

—

Melissa developed shortness of breath at the top of a small hill that led to her job in San Francisco. Otherwise she felt well. Her weight was excellent. Her body mass index, or BMI, of 20 and her waist circumference were normal. She even had her body fat percentage measured by the body pod and found out it was normal at 17%.

She had developed an excellent nutritional program that included eating high-quality foods in the right amount at the right time.

This unexpected shortness of breath sent her to her family doctor.

"What's going on?" Dr. Meredith asked.

"I feel great but I get short of breath climbing a small hill."

"Do you have cough, phlegm, or wheezing?"

"Nothing else, just shortness of breath," Melissa said. "I've never smoked cigarettes and I've never had asthma."

"Does anyone in your family have a lung problem like asthma?"

"No, they're all healthy."

"Do you have any allergies to foods, medicines, or pollens?" Dr. Meredith asked.

"No, nothing."

"Do you have any medical conditions such as diabetes or high blood pressure?"

"No, and I don't take any medicines," Melissa said.

"Hmm, you have crackles when I listen to your lungs," the doctor said.

"What does that mean?" Melissa asked, somewhat worried.

"Let's obtain a chest x-ray to find out."

They reviewed Melissa's chest x-ray and found patchy shadows in both lungs, and a high-resolution chest computer tomography, or CT scan, confirmed the shadows. They were "ground-glass" hazy types, which usually meant inflammation. The shadows had an unusual triangular shape and the open branching airways could be seen in them. This had the appearance of a lung disease called bronchiolitis obliterans organizing pneumonia, or BOOP.

A small lung biopsy was obtained that confirmed the diagnosis. This disease is an inflammatory process and not a scarring process, so prednisone, a powerful anti-inflammatory medicine that would result in complete resolution, was given.

In the meantime, Melissa asked Dr. Meredith: "What caused the BOOP?"

"It's usually called idiopathic BOOP, which means there is no known or associated cause," the doctor said. "Sometimes, though, it's caused by respiratory infections or immune-dysfunction disorders, "but, you didn't have an infection and you don't have any connective tissue disorders."

"What else would cause it?"

"Surprisingly, there are more than 35 medications that can cause BOOP, but you're not taking any of them."

"I'm not taking medicines, but I'm taking a supplement from the health store," Melissa said. "It's called L-tryptophan, used as a sleep aid and for pain relief."

"A standard amount of this generally doesn't cause any problem," Dr. Meredith said. "How much do you take?"

"I might've overdone it," Melissa said cautiously, feeling somewhat embarrassed. "I thought that if a little was good, more would be better. So, I've been taking 2.5 grams every day for the past three months."

"You're right to feel a little uneasy," Dr. Meredith said. "That's ten times higher than the usual dose and it probably caused the BOOP."

"What's going to happen to me? Am I going to die?"

"No, you're not going to die," the doctor reassured her. "The BOOP is moderately severe, but it was found early enough, so it'll respond to treatment and not leave a permanent injury or scar."

"That's a relief," Melissa said.

Melissa stopped taking the tryptophan and soon stopped the prednisone for the BOOP, which quickly improved and completely resolved in a few weeks. She had an excellent diet and exercise program, so Melissa did not need to take extra vitamins or supplements, as they were found in abundant amounts in the healthy foods.

———

Be sure to tell your doctor about all the vitamins and supplements you may be taking, in addition to prescription medications.

An important step in taking a nutritional inventory is documenting your current eating habits – what types of foods you eat, how much you eat, and when you eat.

At the end of the questioning, you'll be asked about occupational or environmental exposures. A helpful way to answer the questions is to begin with your place and date of birth; what you did during the summers; if you had any exposures during school or at home; what your first job involved, including the title and job description. The questions will continue with a review of your chronological list of jobs and potential specific exposures, such as accidental fume exposure, ongoing fume or chemical exposure, and exposure to toxic dusts such as asbestos, beryllium, or silica. You'll be asked about your office air environment. If you had an exposure, how much was the exposure? When did it occur?

———

The second component, after you've answered the questions, is a physical examination. Your vital signs, which include your height, weight, blood pressure, pulse, temperature, respiratory rate, and oxygen saturation, will be obtained. The body mass index (BMI), waist circumference, and body fat percentage will be determined for evaluation of your nutritional status.

Your eyes will be examined for vascular effects of hypertension and diabetes. Your neck and tops of your shoulders will be felt to determine if any lymph nodes are enlarged. The stethoscope will be used to listen to the lungs for wheezing and crackles, and to the heart for murmurs and extra sounds. Your abdomen will be palpated for liver or spleen enlargement. The lower extremities will be evaluated for arthritis, vascular dysfunction, and swelling in the ankles that might represent edema, or fluid.

———

You're ready for the third component – diagnostic testing – and it's time for you to ask questions.

Be sure to ask about the tests and procedures. What are they for? How specific are they? What's the success rate of the tests? Will they be useful for finding a diagnosis specifically for you? What are the risks? Innocuous-appearing tests may have a dark side. False positives can send you down the road to potentially dangerous tests.

Screening tests for nutrition-related diseases include the complete blood count, or CBC, which is information about your white blood cells and red blood cells. It will show whether you have anemia, which could be small red blood cells for iron-deficiency anemia or large red blood cells for folic acid or vitamin B_{12} deficiency. Your electrolyte values will be determined for sodium to tell you about your hydration or loss of sodium from diuretic medications. The electrolytes include determinations of the levels of potassium, uric acid, magnesium, and phosphorous. Glucose will be determined for evaluation of the metabolic syndrome and diabetes.

Organ-specific tests such as kidney and liver function tests will be obtained. Sometimes rheumatological screening tests will be obtained. Cancer screening tests will be obtained.

The blood lipid profile is an important part of defining your nutritional status. Remember that proteins in the blood are transporters – they transport medicines and iron. They also transport fats and cholesterol, and they're called lipoproteins. The blood level can be measured. This panel of tests includes total cholesterol; low-density lipoprotein, or LDL; high-density lipoprotein, or HDL; and triglycerides.

The less dense the lipoproteins, the more fat they carry, and it's the low-density fat carrying lipoproteins (LDL) that can cause inflammation in the internal arterial wall. This can turn into plaque, causing decreased or stopped blood flow, especially in the coronary arteries that provide oxygen for your heart. If the blood stops in these small arteries, you'll have a heart attack.

The very-low-density lipoproteins (VLDL) carry the most fat and it's in the form of *triglycerides*. They carry the trigs from the liver to the fat tissue. The problem is they're in the blood while carrying them and at high levels these fatty lipoproteins can directly injure the internal walls of the arteries. VLDL levels are difficult to measure directly, but they can give you useful information, and by reducing your triglyceride level, you also reduce your VLDL level.

Plaques and fatty deposits also occur in the walls of the arteries leading to the brain. A majority of strokes are due to these plaque-containing arteries leading to the brain as the arteries close off, resulting in death of brain cells.

High triglyceride blood levels are just as dangerous as the low-density lipoproteins, but for a different reason. They cause stressed cells to secrete cytokine, or toxic substances, that directly cause inflamed internal artery walls and accelerate the naturally occurring tiny inflammation points at the branches of the arteries.

There is helpful news. High-density lipoproteins, or HDL, are the good ones. They collect fatty substances from the body's tissues and bring them back to the liver. Not only that, as they bumble along the blood stream, they bind and absorb toxic molecules and eliminate them. The higher the level, the better it protects you from rigid arteries and arterial plaques. Daily exercise is a good way to increase your levels of HDL, and surprisingly, fiber also can increase this protective molecule.

New lipoprotein and triglyceride tests are being developed that may more accurately diagnose increased risk of coronary artery plaque and a heart attack. These tests are being researched to determine their significance, and they may be expensive, but some of them eventually could replace cholesterol level as better predictors.

Determining the homocysteine level can be used as a heart disease risk test. This is an amino acid naturally produced by metabolism. Normal levels are healthy, but high levels of this substance can cause inflamed arteries and blood vessel plaques. If the level is high, it's a helpful test for monitoring. Begin a nutritional program that eliminates inflammation-causing foods, monitor the homocysteine level, and a return to a healthy level can be used to define success. As we mentioned in previous chapters, foods and vegetables containing folic acid, B_6, and B_{12} will help maintain a healthy homocysteine level.

What are some of the other tests? Lipoprotein-a may more accurately diagnose the inherited heart-attack risk trait. Lipoprotein-associated phospholipase, or Lp-PLA$_2$, is an enzyme secreted from inflamed arterial walls. So, if a test of this enzyme is high, it means active inflammation and fatty arterial deposits.

There are different sizes and numbers of the LDL particles. The small LDL particles can pierce the arterial lining and form plaque, while the large particles bounce off the internal artery walls, causing no damage.

High-density lipoprotein subfractions are being studied, and ten subfractions have been identified. The large high-density lipoproteins such as HDL_2 are good protectors of arterial plaque formation, while the small $HDL_{7\text{-}10}$ subclasses may be harmful by causing arterial inflammation.

The bad-quantity carbs pop up here again because high-glycemic foods like sugar and sugary-processed foods and drinks not only cause high blood sugar levels and insulin surge triggering fat storage and increased fatty triglyceride levels, they cause a decrease in the protective HDL level. In addition, the recurrent insulin surges caused by these foods eventually can cause pancreas fatigue and decreased insulin production resulting in high blood sugar levels and diabetes.

Several other diagnostic tests are used for heart disease, hypertension, and diabetes.

Heart disease associated with being overweight includes coronary artery disease from rigid artery walls with plaques that limit oxygen to the heart muscle, causing a heart attack. Peripheral vascular disease of the legs also occurs from the same rigid artery walls in the legs and poor circulation. A stroke can occur from an abnormal heart rhythm such as atrial fibrillation because blood clots in the heart make their way through the blood vessels to the brain.

An echocardiogram is a helpful test for evaluation of the heart valves as well as the function and pressures in the left and right sides of the heart. An exercise stress test is used to detect an abnormal heart rhythm and decreased oxygen delivery to the heart. Sometimes a cardiac catheterization is needed to visualize the coronary arteries.

Causes of hypertension include excess weight, a family background, a kidney disorder, or even an adrenal gland tumor.

Screening kidney tests can be helpful to determine whether to obtain an abdominal ultrasound scan of the kidneys or an abdominal CT scan. Hypertension can cause strokes. If there are neurological symptoms, a magnetic resonance imaging scan, or MRI, of the brain will be obtained.

For diabetes, the "casual" blood glucose concentration is a good start. This means obtaining a blood sample at any time of the day without regard to the last meal. Typical diabetic symptoms and a value of 200 or more is an indication of diabetes.

A fasting blood glucose test can be helpful. This means no caloric intake for at least eight hours, and a value of more than 125 is consistent with diabetes.

The final test is a glucose-tolerance test. This is performed by drinking 75 grams of glucose dissolved in water and measuring the blood glucose level two hours later. A value of 200 or more is diagnostic of diabetes.

The metabolic syndrome is the most common weight-related disorder and the frequency is increasing every day. It's defined as having any one of these conditions: waist measurement of 40 inches or more for men and 35 inches or more for women; triglyceride of 150 or above; high-density lipoprotein, or HDL, cholesterol below 40 for men and below 50 for women; blood pressure of 130/85 or above; or a fasting blood glucose of 100 or above.

There are two types of diabetes. The traditional insulin-dependent diabetes is called type 1 diabetes and results from the pancreas making little or no insulin. Type 2 diabetes is more common and results from insulin resistance in which the body no longer responds to insulin in a normal way.

Pre-diabetes is defined as a fasting blood sugar level between 100 and 125. People with pre-diabetes have an increased risk of type 2 diabetes and are at increased risk for cardiovascular diseases. The type 2 diabetes risk, however, can be decreased for people with pre-diabetes who are able to lose 5% to 7% of their body weight.

Obstructive sleep apnea, or OSA, can be a serious weight-related disorder. Men who have a neck size larger than 17 inches and women who have a neck size larger than 15 inches are at increased risk. This sleep disorder is defined as breathing that stops and starts while a person is sleeping. The breathing may stop for ten seconds or for longer than 30 seconds, and is accompanied by a loud grunting noise opening the airway when the breathing starts again. Snoring is often associated with this sleep disorder.

Observation by a spouse or an observer is the initial diagnostic step. "My husband or my wife stops breathing at night" is a common comment.

Other symptoms include sleep-deprivation symptoms such as falling asleep within a few minutes while sitting or during a conversation with someone. Irritability and lack of concentration are secondary symptoms. If severe, the heart can become enlarged and dysfunctional, and increased vascular pressure may develop in the lungs, referred to as pulmonary hypertension.

———

Paul, 50, was an energetic truck driver who experienced a life-threatening event that sent him to see Dr. Dave Norton.

"So, what's going on, Paul?" Dr. Norton asked.

"I was driving my rig outside of town and remember being at the top of the hill, and I remember being at the bottom of the hill, but I don't remember anything in between," Paul said. "I turned off the truck and had someone drive me home."

"Whoa, you're a wise man," the doctor said with concern. "Let's find out what happened."

"It's been going on for a while; I keep falling asleep during the day," Paul said. "I fall asleep after sitting in a chair for a couple of minutes and even fall asleep talking. I'm really sluggish all day and never feel like I get enough sleep. It makes me cranky and depressed."

"What about sleeping at night? What happens?"

"I go to bed and quickly fall asleep, but find myself waking up after a few minutes, fall asleep, wake up, fall asleep; this happens all night long."

A physical examination showed that Paul was a stocky man with extra weight in his abdomen. His neck size was 18 inches. The lungs and heart were normal.

"You probably have obstructive sleep apnea," Dr. Norton said. "Let's obtain a sleep study to confirm the diagnosis."

Paul underwent a polysomnography study, which meant that he slept overnight in a laboratory in which his breathing, chest and abdominal motion, heart rate, brain-wave activity, eye movements, and oxygen were monitored. It might seem impossible to sleep in these conditions, but people with obstructive sleep apnea are so sleep-deprived, they quickly fall asleep. The apnea and hypopnea episodes are counted. Apnea means breathing has stopped for ten seconds or more, and hypopnea means a 50% decrease in airflow for ten seconds or more.

The study showed that Paul had typical obstructive sleep apnea. His apnea-hypopnic index was 28 per hour. Normal is none to five. In healthy people, the blood oxygen value remains normal above 90% during the night. Not for Paul: his oxygen was less than 90% for 20% of his sleep time and decreased below 75% on three occasions.

"The test confirmed it," Dr. Norton said. "You have obstructive sleep apnea."

"Now what?" Paul asked.

"There are several options. Let's talk about them."

The diagnostic process had been completed. Paul's treatment options will be outlined in the next chapter. You might be surprised. There are always options.

———

It's time to learn more about the diagnostic process involved with Kate and her son. She had weakness and fatigue, and her son had an intermittent upset stomach.

"Kate," Dr. Whatling said, "although your weight is borderline increased, let's do some morphometric measurements to have a more accurate picture of your nutritional status. I'll have the nutritionist meet with you."

"Sounds good to me," she replied.

"You're 5 feet 5 inches and weigh 150 pounds," the nutritionist told Kate, "which makes the body mass index, or BMI, 25. That's at the over-weight mark because 18.5 to 24.9 is in the healthy range and obesity is more than 30."

"That's what I was afraid of," Kate said. "The weight came on during pregnancy, and I didn't take the effort needed to return to my healthy weight. But that doesn't seem like it's high enough to cause this feeling of being tired?"

"Let's check a couple of other measurements," the nutritionist said. "We'll measure your waist measurement at your belly button and upper hip bone. The BMI (body mass index) might be high in athletes because of increased muscle mass, but the waist circumference will be normal in these athletes. Your waist is 35 inches, also right at the high-risk level. The risks include type 2 diabetes, hypertension, and coronary artery disease."

"Now you're scaring me," Kate said.

"No reason for alarm," the nutritionist said calmly. "It's borderline, so it can be fixed, but that still doesn't tell us why you're weak and fatigued."

"Let's do one more measurement."

Kate's fat percentage was measured with the air displacement method in a body pod available in the laboratory. The water-displacement may be considered the most accurate, but it's not routinely available and takes too much time. Other methods include skin calipers or body measure-ment calculations. There is also an easy electronic hand-held machine available. These methods are less accurate, but easy to do and helpful for monitoring purposes.

"We found the answer," the nutritionist said. "Your body-fat percent-age is 38%. That's high and in the obesity level. It's usually 15% for women athletes and 25% for healthy women."

"Is that causing my fatigue?" Kate asked

"Yes, that's the cause. Too much stored fat can cause sluggishness. Because of the sedentary lifestyle of so many people, there's a name for this finding. It's not flattering, but it's called the 'metabolically obese.' People are not obese by weight measurements, but they are by metabolic measurements."

"Your blood tests also showed that your iron level is borderline low."

"Amazing," Kate said. "I never thought that eating the wrong types of foods could cause so much trouble."

"Yes, but the situation can be corrected," the nutritionist said. "It's making some changes in food choices and amounts."

The management options for Kate will be outlined in the next chapter.

———

Kate talked to Dr. Whaling about her son.

"He seems to be having digestive symptoms," Kate said. "Sometimes he has abdominal pain on the right side, and he says he feels like his stomach is bloated, but I'm not sure what he means."

"It could be appendicitis," Dr. Whatling said.

"These are intermittent symptoms with no sudden onset of the pain in the lower right side," Kate said, "and he doesn't have a fever."

"No, that doesn't sound like acute appendicitis, but irritable bowel syndrome, or IBS, is a consideration."

"What's IBS?"

"It's a strange name but irritable bowel syndrome is a crabby colon that causes alternating constipation and diarrhea," Dr. Whatling said. "Symptoms also include cramps and bloating like your son described."

"This could be it, but isn't he too young to have this?"

"Yes, IBS usually occurs during ages 25 to 50, and it occurs more commonly among women.

"How's his mood? These symptoms may occur in people who are depressed."

"Oh, he's fantastic," Kate said. "He's an active guy and captain of the football team."

"What about his diet? Are there any foods that bother him?"

By now, Craig had joined his mother in the doctor's office. "I seem to have trouble after eating cereal," Craig told the doctor.

"Hmm, it could be gluten intolerance," Dr. Whatling said.

"Sounds really strange. What's gluten?" Craig asked.

"Gluten is a protein found in wheat, barley, and rye," the doctor said. "It actually means glue, and is the chewy substance in these products that give them shape. Some people are allergic to wheat and some people have celiac disease, which is a genetic-based immune reaction to gliadin, one of the constituents of gluten, with the other being glutelin. The immune dysfunction causes inflammation, resulting in damage to the small intestine villi, tiny tubular projections from the intestinal wall needed for nutrient absorption, which become flattened and unable to function well."

"That's a long explanation; so what's next?" Craig asked.

"Let's try a different diagnostic approach. Instead of obtaining blood tests and x-rays, let's try an exclusionary diet, which means you eliminate gluten-containing foods to see if the symptoms go away."

Kate and Craig learned about foods that contain gluten and began carefully reading food labels. Craig began a diet that contained no gluten and all symptoms disappeared after two weeks. Later, the diagnosis of celiac disease was confirmed with laboratory studies. The standard has been a biopsy of the small intestine, but anti-gliadin antibody tests have been a big advance in the diagnosis.

———

They understood the diagnostic process, and can now hear about their treatment options. That's the third vital step. Know your treatment options, which we'll learn about in the next chapter.

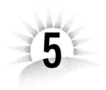

5

Plenty of Treatment Options:
Diet Pills, Bypass, Weight-loss Programs, the Epler Health Plan

It's time to learn about your treatment options for nutrition-related disorders. What are the options for weight loss? And what are the treatment options for diseases that are related to being overweight?

Weight-loss treatment options

You know your desired healthy weight, and you're over that mark. Many options exist that can get you to your desired goal, so many that you can become overwhelmed and give up. But one of those options is best for you.

Learn the benefits of each option. Learn the science. Does it make sense? Learn about the risks, and especially the long-term risks over several years. Overnight solutions usually are not best for you. You're searching for a long-term nutrition plan with flexibility that will adapt to your changing nutrition needs over time, to new information about nutrition, and to new food choices. Patience is key during this process.

You should be aware of a couple of factors as you begin a weight-loss program. During the first week, you'll lose weight, but it's water weight;

the losses during the next three weeks probably would be from muscle mass. Surprisingly, it's not until week four that you begin to lose fat. From there, it's going to take additional effort.

You will need to burn up 3,500 calories to lose one pound of fat and that's on top of your basal metabolic needs. This means that if you eat 500 fewer calories each day, that pound will come off in a week. That's 50 pounds in a year—more than enough to solve your overall problem.

An additional subtle but important part about weight loss is that, as you lose weight, you'll require fewer calories. For example, if you lose 20 pounds, the loss of the second 10 is going to be slower than the first 10. Furthermore, if you continue to consume the same number of calories, the weight loss eventually will stop because the number of calories will equal the amount of energy consumed.

Let's consider a common cosmetic issue. What can you do about the extra pounds of belly fat? The belly has grown larger gradually over the years. You don't like it and it doesn't look good.

It'll be harder than you think to make it shrink.

Start by learning everything you can about increased belly fat. Too much high-glycemic carbohydrates and processed foods, such as white starchy foods, is a major cause, along with a subconscious habit of eating more food than you need. The quantity of food is just too high—you take in too much food to burn as energy and the left over turns to fat.

Specifically, the excess glucose that is not burned is converted into fat deposition in the middle. A small amount of the right type of long-chain carbohydrates is a good source of long-term energy without triggering insulin spikes and fat deposition. But excess amounts will turn quickly into belly fat, and it doesn't take much.

Chronic or repeated stress is a contributor because it releases cortisol, causing increased blood sugar, which is not burned completely, and the remaining turns to midsection fat. This is why, if you're stressed, taking three to five belly breaths before eating will improve digestion. In addition, ask yourself if you're eating something to relieve stress; if so, this food will turn into midsection fat.

You'll learn that abdominal-core exercises can make up an important part of the maintenance of a slim belly, but, by themselves, they will not decrease belly fat. It's important to do them correctly. Learn them from a good personal trainer. Abdominal-core exercises need to be performed when the stomach is flat, not crunched toward the chest.

Liposuction is an option that you can discuss with your doctor. It's important to ask questions about the long-term benefits and risks. Ask questions until you truly understand the answers. What will your stomach look like in ten years? One issue is that when you regain fat deposits, they may appear in an irregular pattern of lumps and bumps, and will look worse than a smooth, rounded belly. Ask questions. Find out if the risk is worth the benefit.

So, how will you lose that midsection weight? It's up to you. Have a good attitude. You *can* lose it. Learn everything you can. Eat the right type of high-quality foods in the right amounts.

——

What are the management options for someone who is dangerously overweight and at increased risk of developing obesity-related, life-threatening diseases? The options include physician-directed diet pills, surgical procedures, special diets, weight-loss programs, and the development of your own plan.

Diet pills

Taking diet pills can be an appealing approach because it's easy and can be effective. But the short- and long-term effects can be deadly and must be fully considered.

In the past, a prescribed combination of pills was utilized that resulted in significant weight loss in many individuals, but the price was too high for a small number of people. A complication developed that took their lives. The pills were taken off the market.

Are there safe diet-pill options? That depends on many factors. Over-the-counter, weight-loss pills that you can purchase at the drug store, supermarket, or health store are for people who wish to lose a few pounds. It's important to be aware that these pills are not subject to the rigorous federal drug approval process for efficacy and safety, but the Federal Drug Administration, or FDA, monitors these agents once they are on the shelf and will ban them, if necessary. That leaves you in charge of learning about them.

Read the label carefully and talk to the pharmacist about a medication you're considering. Purchase the pills from a company with high manufacturing standards so there will be no impurities and the dose will be accurate; sometimes the drug contains only a fraction of the dose listed on the label.

Prescription drugs that have been approved for over-the-counter use have been thoroughly tested, but again, review the drug manufacturing company to ensure that the product is pure and the dosage is accurate. Then, read the label for adverse reactions such as liver injury because a doctor or nurse will not be monitoring your usage.

In rare situations, deceitful companies will add substances to their products and not list them on the label; for example, they'll market a multivitamin product as a muscle-building product, when that product unlawfully contains an anabolic steroid. FDA websites can be helpful in detecting such companies, addressing safety concerns, and monitoring potential product recalls.

Prescription diet pills are generally limited to people who have a major overweight condition and who have complications such as diabetes or hypertension. In these situations, it's recommended that pills be taken in conjunction with nutrition management and exercise programs in partnership with your physician team. Unless a person has developed a long-term, nutrition-management program, excess weight will return as soon as the medication is stopped.

Gastric bypass

The most common type of gastric-bypass surgery is the Roux-en-Y gastric bypass, named after a Swiss surgeon, Dr. César Roux.

The stomach is divided into two parts. A new, small, upper "pouch" stomach is formed and food goes directly to the small intestine. Food no longer goes to the larger, remaining stomach. This limits the amount of food that can be eaten and results in weight loss.

Most medical centers have established rigorous criteria that must be met before individuals can undergo this procedure. The criteria may include a body-mass index, or BMI, of 40 or more, which is extreme obesity; or weight-related health problems such as hypertension, cardiovascular disease, or diabetes for individuals with a lower BMI.

The next step is to meet with a surgeon, internist, nutritionist, and a psychologist. This review includes eating habits, degree of exercise, smoking history, and alcohol use.

You will have several baseline laboratory studies that are used to monitor long-term adverse reactions. The psychological evaluation includes your stress level, motivation, binge-eating pattern, substance abuse, depression, or anxiety disorders. The surgery is delayed if issues requiring correction are discovered.

Learn about the benefits. Most individuals quickly lose weight after the procedure and lose weight for the first year. They can lose up to 80% of their excess weight in four to five years. The feeling of being full is derived from stretch receptors in the stomach wall, so with a smaller stomach, the feeling occurs with a smaller amount of food.

In addition to this weight loss, the procedure may improve or resolve several obesity-related disorders, including type-2 diabetes, high blood pressure, and high blood cholesterol and lipid levels, all of which would decrease the risks of having a heart attack or stroke.

In the last chapter, Paul learned that weight loss could improve or eliminate obstructive sleep apnea. It may decrease gastroesophageal reflux disease, or GERD. It improves leg swelling and associated venous disease that is often associated with obesity. Lower back pain along with knee pain often can be relieved or improved. Weight loss improves the quality of life. It's easier to get around, be active, and avoid shortness of breath.

But, know the risks of gastric-bypass surgery. Short-term complications range from 5% to 15%, which can include anesthesia difficulties, infection at the incision site, leaking of the stomach contents into the abdominal cavity, bleeding into the abdomen or into the bowel, ulcers, and blood clots in the lungs. Some of these complications may be monitored through observation or treated with antibiotics, transfusions, and in some situations, another surgery. The risk of death, which may occur at one to two per 1,000, is associated with this surgery.

Some patients may develop recurrent vomiting after surgery that can lead to protein deficiency, and protein supplements can be helpful during this period.

It's important to know not only the postoperative risks, but to know what to expect during the postoperative period to minimize the effects. For example, transient muscle weakness and balancing problems may occur, and knowing about these possibilities prior to surgery can be helpful.

Emotional and psychological effects may occur during the three-month, postoperative period. Depression and low energy levels may occur because food may have played a big role in the past and people need to develop lifestyle changes to fulfill this role. Reviewing these issues with the nutrition psychologist beforehand can be useful.

Long-term complications can include hernias, which are openings through muscles. They may develop at the abdominal incision site or internally. Small bowel obstructions may occur from internal scarring or adhesions from the surgery. This obstruction can trap the bowel, cutting off the blood supply, which often requires surgical repair. About one-third of people may develop gallstones, anemia, or osteoporosis.

Nutritional and metabolic deficiencies are important long-term considerations. Iron deficiency may be a serious deficiency because normally iron is absorbed in the duodenum, which is bypassed in the Roux-en-Y gastric-bypass procedure. Supplemental iron tablets can be used, or in severe situations, injections of iron can be given.

Vitamin B_{12} deficiency causes a different type of anemia, called macrocytic anemia, because the red blood cells are larger than normal. This vitamin requires intrinsic factor from the cells lining the stomach, so with a smaller stomach, an insufficient amount of vitamin B_{12} may be absorbed. This deficiency also may cause neuropathy, which is dysfunctional nerves, resulting in numbness and weakness. Supplemental vitamin B_{12} tablets or liquid taken under the tongue, or sublingual, may be sufficient. Once-monthly injections may be required.

Calcium deficiency can be a problem after a gastric bypass. Calcium is absorbed in the duodenum, which is bypassed by surgery, and that means no absorption, resulting in low blood calcium and bone loss. Low calcium causes hyperparathyroidism. The small parathyroid glands are located along the thyroid gland in the neck, and the parathyroid hormones regulate calcium. If the calcium is low, the parathyroid makes more parathyroid hormone, which can cause osteoporosis, fatigue, and sometimes depression.

Life-threatening abnormal cardiac rhythm can occur with severe hypocalcemia. Supplemental vitamin D and calcium can manage this situation, and because of the bypassed duodenum, the type of calcium can make a difference: Calcium citrate is better than calcium carbonate.

Can this type of gastric surgery be reversed? Surgeons who perform the Roux-en-Y bypass generally consider the surgery permanent because of the major stomach and intestinal structural changes that are made. Theoretically, the changes can be reversed, but there is risk. It's important to discuss this issue with your surgeon prior to undergoing the procedure.

Diets

This type of weight-loss management means eating specified types and amounts of foods as directed by a predetermined formula or set of instructions, usually for a limited length of time. As with all weight-loss methods, learn the benefits and risks. Most are safe but others can be risky, especially in the long term.

An extreme emotional element is associated with dieting, so people are subject to peer pressure and advertising. Some of the diets become so popular that people feel guilty because they're not using them. They can be effective in the short term, but if a long-term nutrition plan has not been developed, the pounds can return quickly when the diet is stopped. It's important to remember that people gain more weight the second and third time they stop; strangely enough, diets can cause people to gain weight.

Despite these considerations, each of the diets may have good features that can provide helpful information for nutrition management. For example, the use of olive oil from the Mediterranean diet instead of highly saturated fat cooking oils is a positive finding. The Sonoma diet controls portion sizes. The helpful feature of the DASH diet for hypertension is a way to decrease sodium intake to safe levels. The South Beach diet emphasizes eating low-glycemic carbohydrates—the vegetables and foods that do not cause an insulin surge and the fat storage response. The Paleolithic, or Stone Age, diet sounds like an unlikely success, but eating nonprocessed food and locally grown fruits and vegetables is healthy.

Review them intensely. One may be the right approach for you.

Weight-loss programs

This type of weight-loss management involves joining a weight-loss program that may or may not include purchases of prepared foods. These programs have been successful for some people, especially because people learn about the psychological issues of eating and learn to develop a lifelong program.

As with pills and diets, learn about the benefits and learn about the risks. Read the labels of purchased foods. Just because they are sold by a healthy weight-loss program doesn't mean they're healthy. Look out for high sugar and sodium content. These programs can be expensive, and once the program is stopped, the weight can return quickly and sometimes more than the pre-diet baseline.

Some of these programs have good features.

For example, Weight-Watchers® has been around for decades, and the strength is utilizing the power of group support, and it has kept up with changes in science and social media. Members can attend local meetings or join the online program.

Nutrisystem® is a program that has portion-controlled meals that can be delivered; the plan, if followed correctly, allows calorie control.

Study all the programs. One of them may work for you. Internet-based weight-loss programs have been shown to be helpful for some people, and be sure to read about the benefits and risks.

The Epler Health Diet Plan

This approach is a guide to your own lifelong nutrition management. It's based on continually learning everything you can about nutrition that applies to you. It means constantly adjusting the types and the amounts of foods you eat as new information about foods and new foods become available. It means having a healthy mind.

The plan gives you a framework to put food to work for you:

- Eat high-quality foods in the right amounts at the right time and place.
- Exercise regularly and maintain healthy sleep.
- Keep a positive attitude, because you're the one in charge.

That's the plan, and here it is in more detail.

High-quality foods are those grown as close as possible to nature, such as fruits and vegetables grown in fields that are maintained by hand. These include U.S. government green-label organic foods. High-quality foods are not multi-ingredient processed foods that you reheat for dinner. High-quality foods contain no added sodium or salt, and no added sugar.

High-quality meats include chicken and beef from free-range animals not given supplemental substances or hormones, and likewise with high-quality dairy. High-quality seafood comes from fish living free in the ocean, lakes, or rivers.

Add in healthy carbohydrates such as whole grains and colorful fruits and vegetables that do not cause an insulin surge, triglyceride spikes, and fat deposition. Avoid and keep to a minimum low threshold carbohydrates like sugar, sugary foods and drinks, foods like pastries, candies, and ice cream. Eliminate foods containing trans fat. Avoid and keep to a minimum low threshold fats like fatty meats, bacon and processed meats like hot dogs and sausages. Maintain a healthy omega-6/omega-3 balance, keeping the omega-3 fatty acids at a high level. Eat foods containing soluble and insoluble fiber.

As you choose among foods at the supermarket or restaurant, select foods and quantities that are safe, foods that have anti-inflammatory activity, and foods that can neutralize toxic substances. For example, one-half of an avocado has two grams of palmitic acid, the potentially bad-quantity saturated fatty acid, but has nine grams of oleic acid, the monounsaturated fat, and two grams of linoleic acid, the polyunsaturated fatty acid. Therefore, both of the healthy fatty acids outweigh the saturated fatty acid. In addition, avocado has potassium to counteract too much sodium from other foods, both magnesium and manganese to maintain soft and pliable arteries, and fiber for neutralizing toxic substances. However, the omega-6/omega-3 ratio is too high at 15, so balance is needed—this ratio will need to be reduced by adding a high omega-3 food.

For individuals with extreme obesity and complications such as cardiovascular disease and diabetes, partner actively with a physician team to develop a safe and successful weight-loss program.

The plan includes copying the characteristics of people who live beyond the age of 100. They are the vigorous centenarians and there are more of them than ever before.

Exercise and walk regularly. Take the stairs whenever you can. Use the 20-minute imperative—exercise 20 minutes every day for health—more for additional benfits. Maintain a healthy weight and minimize foods with saturated fats such as burgers, minimize sugar by not drinking sodas or sugary beverages, minimize sodium and salt use, and consume purple fruits and vegetables. Obvious traits of the centenarians include no use of tobacco or excessive use of alcohol.

Floss. It's surprising advice, but people who have lived past 100 have flossed, which prevents gum disease and chronic inflammation that could lead to oral cancers. These centenarians don't sleep too much or too little. They have healthy minds—they're optimistic. They have upbeat friends and constantly seek new challenges.

You can, too. Your nutrition balance, and your health, is in your hands.

Obesity-related disease treatment options

Diabetes: Insulin is usually needed for type 1 diabetes, while weight loss may improve or eliminate type 2 diabetes. If they are deemed necessary, several types of medicines are used for the treatment of type 2 diabetes.

Hypertension: There are several different types of hypertension. The most common is called essential hypertension, from an unknown cause. Keeping sodium intake to a minimum is fundamental management. This type usually requires medications, which begin with mild antihypertensive pills that are titrated, or increased, to stronger medications and higher doses until the hypertension is controlled.

There are no symptoms from hypertension except for an extreme hypertensive crisis, so you need to take the medication even though you don't feel any effects. This is a reason blood pressure monitoring with a home blood pressure cuff is so useful. It can tell you whether the medicine is helping. You should ask about the side effects of the specific pills you're taking, especially ten-year, long-term side effects, as these medicines are prescribed for many years.

Diagnostic tests may confirm other types of hypertension, such as from arterial malformation, kidney dysfunction, or hormone imbalance. These types are treated with surgery or hormone replacement. Ask about the treatment options and risks.

Overweight-related hypertension can be improved or eliminated by returning to a healthy weight. Low sodium and salt intake is an important part of overweight-related hypertension.

Heart disease, kidney disease, and eye disease: Coronary artery disease, which means atherosclerotic plaques in the arteries supplying blood to the heart, can be prevented by eating heart-healthy foods that have no or low-saturated fat, no trans fat, no or low sugar and sodium, low-glycemic foods, and high-fiber foods. Type 2 diabetes and weight-gain hypertension can cause cardiovascular disease, kidney disease, and eye disease. Maintenance of a healthy weight can prevent these conditions.

Obstructive sleep apnea: Weight loss can improve and even eliminate this condition in some individuals. The neck size decreases and the muscles that maintain an open trachea become more effective. There are several other treatment options.

———

Remember Paul? He had severe sleep deprivation and potentially harmful consequences from his obstructive sleep apnea. He and Dr. Norton discussed his treatment.

"For people with obstructive sleep apnea, the soft muscle at the back of the throat is weak and flaccid, resulting in closing off the trachea or windpipe when lying flat," the doctor explained. "So, sleeping on your side can be helpful."

"What else?" Paul asked.

"There are mechanical devices that can keep open the airways, and some surgeons have developed an operation.

"For you, CPAP may be the best option."

"Sounds strange, what's CPAP?"

"The letters stand for continuous positive airway pressure. It's a fitted face mask that delivers a small amount of pressure each time you take a breath, keeping the airway open all night."

"I have to sleep with a mask and a noisy machine?"

"Yes, it sounds difficult, but people all over the world use the treatment. It's really helpful. It allows you to regain your energy so that you can accomplish the best treatment—losing weight."

"You mean losing weight will resolve the situation?"

"Yes, sometimes just 20 pounds, but getting to your healthy weight is best."

"That's a tall order," Paul said, "but I'm going to have to do it because this sleep apnea is dangerous.

"Before I get fitted for CPAP, I wanted to tell you that I strained my neck and would like a neck brace."

"Sure, not a problem," Dr. Norton said as he wrote an order for a neck brace.

Paul returned to the doctor two weeks later. Dr. Norton was surprised and amazed when Paul walked into the office. He swaggered as if he were walking onto a Broadway stage—head up and a big smile.

"You look fantastic. What'd you do?" the doctor asked.

"Well, Doc, I wore that neck collar you gave me at night and slept all night long," Paul replied enthusiastically. "I was full of energy the next day!"

"Hmm, this may be a new treatment."

"It worked for me," Paul said. "I know it's only short term, but it's giving me plenty of energy to lose that 20 pounds you talked about and eventually get back to a healthy weight."

"Sounds good to me, Paul," the doctor said.

———

Know the treatment options for your weight-related disorders and find the one that's best for you.

———

Let's revisit the treatment options for Kate and her son, Craig. Kate was diagnosed with an unusual but common situation called metabolically obese, and Craig had celiac disease.

"Now what should I do?" Kate asked her nutritionist.

"Types of foods are important," the nutritionist said, "but in your situation, it's not only the types but the quantity—you're taking in too many calories, especially from too many processed carbohydrates that are causing the abdominal weight increase."

"What do carbohydrates have to do with fat?" Kate asked.

"At first, carbohydrates are burned up for energy, but if too much is consumed, the leftover causes insulin and cortisol release, which result in fat storage, and that's often in the belly. And too much in the belly is dangerous. It results in the diseases we've talked about, including cardiovascular disease, hypertension, and type 2 diabetes."

"You convinced me; too much carbohydrate can turn to fat," Kate said. "So, what are the good ones and bad ones?"

"It's not so much good or bad, it's the quantity threshold that counts," the nutritionist said. "The good-quantity ones are whole grains, vegetables, legumes, fiber, and fruits. Fresh vegetables grown locally, whole foods, and low-ingredient foods are best. The bad-quantity ones? Anything else. Processed and packaged carbohydrates often contain excessive sodium and sugar, often in the form of high-fructose concentrate, making it easy to consume too many calories. Sugary drinks can pack on the abdominal fat quickly. Salt and sugar make foods almost addicting.

You can't stop eating them. Remember, fiber is a good carb—it slows digestion for a steady stream of energy and eliminates insulin surges."

"What about amount of food," Kate asked. "Are there foods that can be eaten in an unlimited amount?"

"That's the quantity threshold I talked about," the nutritionist said. "Some foods need to be eaten in much less quantities than others. For example, baked potatoes have a high glycemic index which means they can cause an insulin and cortisol surge and fat deposition, but if boiled and eaten in a small amount, there is no insulin response. A vegetable like spinach is usually eaten in the right amount and has all types of extra healthy nutrients like iron, folate, omega-3 fatty acids, and manganese."

"Is there anything else wrong with too many bad-quantity carbs?"

"Big problem, it's the unhealthy carbohydrates and too much concentrated fructose that cause a high triglyceride level in your blood, which causes vascular inflammation."

"Whoa," Kate said, "I didn't realize too many of the wrong-quantity carbs can be so dangerous."

"Yes, but you can manage them."

"What about the fats? Should I eliminate them?"

"No, you don't want to do that. You need healthy fats. They're needed to absorb fat-soluble vitamins, build cell structure, and maintain healthy skin. They also have a high appetite-satisfaction index, so you eat less."

"Which ones are healthy?"

"They're the unsaturated fats, either polyunsaturated or monosaturated fatty acids. The polyunsaturated fats include omega-3 fatty acids found in cold-water fish like salmon, and in flaxseed. The monounsaturated fats are found in foods such as olive oil and avocado."

"I can guess the unhealthy ones—they're the saturated ones," Kate said.

"Yup, everyone knows about the saturated fats—keep them at a minimum," the nutritionist said. "There are several of them and they have low-quantity thresholds. For example, palmitic acid is a common saturated fatty acid and it seems to be everywhere, and at low levels it may even be beneficial, but the threshold is low, go over it, and it's hazardous by increasing the low-density lipoproteins in the blood that inflame the artery walls and cause fatty plaques in the coronary arteries, causing a heart attack."

"What are the worse foods?"

"You know most of the culprits—fatty animal and dairy products, especially processed meats and lunch meats. Old-fashioned lard is one of the worst. Read the labels. There's a ton of saturated fats in candy bars and in some chips."

"Eliminating saturated fat sounds impossible?" Kate asked.

"Yes, it's impossible. Fortunately, the body seems to be capable of managing 20 to 25 grams of saturated fat on a daily basis. Over those amounts, they'll increase your blood low-density lipoproteins that injure your arteries."

"Ah, saturated fats cause inflamed arteries. Too much of the wrong type of carbohydrates cause abdominal fat and inflamed arteries," Kate said. "Food sounds dangerous!"

"Oh, no. Food's wonderful," the nutritionist said. "You just need to learn a couple of important things about it and manage it successfully. Put it to work for you. The right food in the right quantity and it'll take care of you."

"What are trans fats?" Kate asked. "I've heard they're bad for the heart."

"You're right. They may be worse than saturated fat because they not only increase the bad low-density lipoproteins, or LDL, but they decrease the good high-density lipoproteins, or HDL.

"The tiny amounts of naturally occurring trans fats in foods are of minimal concern. But there are the artificial trans fats that are manufactured when liquid oils are changed to the solid form, such as found in margarines. These artificial trans fats can also be found in high amounts in fried foods, pastries, processed foods, and some snack foods. Fortunately, because of a recent food labeling requirement, these artificial trans fats have been eliminated in many foods."

"I hear that fried foods are not healthy," Kate said. "How can frying food in a small amount of oil be so unhealthy?"

"That's a good question," the nutritionist said. "I asked that same question during my training, and I quickly learned."

"What's the answer?"

"Fried foods are probably close to the number one source of unhealthy saturated fats in the diet, because it's the saturated fat they're fried in, which seems like a small amount, but these foods are so tasty that huge amounts are consumed," the nutritionist said. "Try eating one french fry or one potato chip. It's impossible. Fried chicken and fried seafood—these are tasty foods and can be eaten in massive quantities."

"You're right. How's it possible to eliminate these foods?"

"Begin by limiting the amount. Then develop a taste for healthy choices, and you'll feel better because you're eating healthier food. This is an interesting concept—you begin eating alternative healthy foods that at first are bland and not exciting, but you say to yourself, it's not going to harm me, which gives you a pleasant feeling. You'll be surprised but this second feeling is stronger than the feeling of satisfaction from eating unhealthy food, and eventually replaces it."

"Sounds like some deep thinking, but I've heard about this idea for breaking bad addictive habits, and it works," Kate replied.

"Yes, it does; try it."

"What about protein? That's all good, isn't it?" Kate asked.

"You're right; just about all protein is healthy," the nutritionist said. "It's the associated food that's the problem. We talked earlier about fried chicken and fried seafood, but the beneficial protein is offset by the hazardous fried saturated fats. Even protein energy bars can have excessive sugar and sodium."

"Are there any other unsuspected saturated fats among the healthy protein?" Kate asked.

"The tastiest, tender steaks are often from pen-raised cattle and marbled with saturated fats."

"So, that's why people make such a big deal about free-range and organic chickens, and free-water, nonfarm fish," Kate said.

"Yes, it makes sense. Penned-in cows, cooped-up chickens, and farm-raised fish that are overfed will have too much saturated fat. Salmon from the ocean or rapidly flowing rivers is the best choice. It's even best to eat cage-free eggs from free-range chickens."

"My friend is a vegetarian and I don't think she eats enough protein," Kate said. "Her immune system is weak and she actually gained weight especially, around the middle. What are sources of healthy protein for her?"

"A diet limited to cheese, salads, and pasta for vegetarians is protein poor, and could be dangerous, leading to a poor immune system, sluggishness, and even shortened height in children."

"Protein sources include whole grains. For example, quinoa is filled with good nutrients. It contains all the essential amino acids, and it also contains a high amount of magnesium, which keeps blood vessels flexible and healthy. It contains no sodium and even contains potassium, which can counteract excessive sodium from other foods. Barley is a good source of protein and has a high amount of fiber, which can help maintain a healthy blood lipid profile."

"What else?"

"Beans are great sources of protein," the nutritionist said. "Soy beans and tofu can be healthy sources of protein, but it's really important to read the labels. Some processed foods such as tofu hot dogs or burgers can have excessive amounts of sodium and contain saturated fats, just as hazardous as traditional hot dogs. Some processed sausages even have sugar in them. Soy sauce can have a huge amount of sodium. The protein is healthy, but your friend needs to pay attention. It may be accompanied by excessive sodium, saturated fats, and even sugar."

"What's tempeh?" Kate asked. "I've heard good things about it."

"It's fermented beans or grains," the nutritionist said. "It may be one of the highest sources of pure protein available with no sodium, saturated fat, or sugar. Whey isolate created from cheese can be a healthy protein for many people."

"These are some great healthy sources of protein for vegetarians and for everyone else, too," Kate said.

"Remember we talked about your borderline low iron level?"

"Yes, I remember," Kate said. "What should I do?"

"Your level is not dangerously low and can be brought into healthy levels by eating the right types of foods, such as spinach and other iron-rich foods. We'll monitor your level to make sure it returns to a healthy value."

"Sounds great," Kate said. "Thanks for your help."

———

It was Craig's turn to learn about his treatment. He asked the nutritionist how to manage his celiac disease.

"Eliminate gluten," the nutritionist said. "This means eliminating all gluten protein in foods. The good news is that completely eliminating gluten, especially gliadin, will stop the inflammation in the small intestine, control the symptoms, and prevent the complications."

"Sounds impossible. What foods do I avoid?" Craig asked.

"Grains are the common ones," the nutritionist said. "These include barley, farina, graham flour, matzo meal, rye, semolina, and wheat. Foods that need to be avoided if they are not labeled as gluten-free include all types of beer, breads, candy, cakes and pies, cookies, cereals, crackers, croutons, gravy, processed meats or seafood, oats, pastas, salad dressings, sauces, and soups. Surprisingly, quinoa can be consumed without difficulty."

"That's a big list and really has some good foods," Craig said.

"Yes, but fortunately, many grocery stores have a gluten-free section and now many foods are labeled gluten-free, so there are still many different types of healthy foods.

"There are also unsuspected products to avoid, including food additives such as malt flavoring, lipsticks or lip balms, binding agents in medications or vitamins, and even some types of toothpaste. It's helpful to use separate cutting boards and take care not to mix bread crumbs with other foods. Among the nongluten foods, remember to eat enough foods rich in iron, calcium, B vitamins, folate, and fiber."

"Now that really sounds impossible," Craig said. "I'm a kid. I'm captain of the football team. I can't do it."

"I'm not telling you it's going to be easy, especially at first," the nutritionist said, "but once you find out the foods to avoid, you'll develop a great list of good-tasting and enjoyable foods so that eventually you won't even think about it."

"I'm going to have another problem," Craig said. "I don't want people to know I need a special diet and can't eat their food, especially when I go to people's houses for dinner or go out to eat with my friends."

"Yes, this could be a problem. Some people become so obsessed with their condition avoiding gluten that they drive people away. You need to have a positive approach to the issue and, over time, you'll find what works for you. Besides, the idea of gluten-free food is becoming so well-known that almost everyone is familiar with it, so I think you'll adapt."

"You're probably right," Craig said. "I need to approach it like winning a football game. I can do this and not turn it into a problem."

———

Kate developed her weight management program and Craig learned how to manage his celiac disorder. In the next chapter, we'll describe how you can monitor your nutrition. Kate's story will continue also, and we'll learn about her two friends who had unusual weight-gain problems.

Monitor Your Progress:
What, When, How Do You Eat

You've learned about nutrition, and now understand the diagnostic process of nutrition-related diseases. And you know the treatment options. Monitoring your nutrition is the next step toward a successful management plan.

Measuring your weight is the easiest and most readily available monitoring procedure. Other measurements include body-mass index (BMI), waist circumference, and percentage of body fat.

Write them down, or better yet, monitor these numbers with your computer. You can color-code them to easily see trends. As part of a weight-loss program, it's also helpful to include two or three mental health monitors. You can choose from eight life-index scores. Here they are—six of them you score from zero to ten including stress level, anger level, depression score, fear level, and worry score—three of them you score from ten to zero including how-much-you-like-yourself score, how often you think in a positive way, and your-satisfaction-with-life score. You can read more about these eight life-index scores in Dr. Epler's book,

You're the Boss: Manage Your Disease. High scores will give you energy to succeed with your plan.

Ask yourself three questions at each monitoring point.

Are you improving, or approaching your goal? If so, stay the course.

Are you the same? Continue your plan and give yourself more time. Repeat the question at the next monitoring point.

Are you worse? Action is usually required. If you have a weight-loss plan, talk to your physician or nutritionist about adjusting your plan. If it's a nutrition-related disease and an emergency, you might have to call 911 or visit the emergency room.

———

Becky's weight had gradually increased to dangerous levels and she had developed type 2 diabetes and hypertension. So, she created a weight-loss program with her doctor and nutritionist. She enjoyed using her computer and had written a color-coded program that had several measurements.

"Let's review your results during the past month," the nutritionist said. "They look good. Your weight has decreased steadily, and there has been a slight decrease in waist circumference. The percent fat is about the same. The diabetes and hypertension have improved slightly. Keep up the good work."

Becky returned the next month with disappointing results.

"There's been no change," the nutritionist said. "What about your exercise markers and your life-index scores?"

"Those are both problems," Becky said. "I only exercised once and my life-index scores decreased."

"What'd you monitor?"

"The depression score, how-much-you-like-yourself score, and your-satisfaction-with-life score."

"Those are good ones, but what happened? They decreased this month?"

"I'm disappointed in myself," Becky said. "I kept saying that I can't do this. It's too much work. I've tried this over and over in the past and failed. I can't exercise. I don't want to deal with discipline."

"Whoa, that type of thinking would destroy any program," the nutritionist said with empathy. "Look at the good things. You didn't go backward. Your diabetes and hypertension didn't worsen. You're still on track."

"You're right, it's not so bad."

"That was then and this is now. Approach the situation in a positive way. Say to yourself that you can succeed and you can follow the plan. Say cancel, cancel, cancel each time one of those negative thoughts pops into your mind, and resume building your confidence."

"You're right," Becky said. "The negative thoughts are doing me in. I'm in charge. I can cancel them."

"Keep trying to exercise every day. It really works," the nutritionist said. "Find someone just like you and work out together. There's power in numbers and you get to support each other."

It was hard work for Becky, but she returned the next month with better numbers in all of her monitors. She was succeeding again. She continued to monitor the measurements, and over a two-year program, her blood pressure returned to a normal range and her type 2 diabetes disappeared. Her health-life index scores were high. She had reached all of her goals.

———

Becky's monitoring system allowed her to regain her confidence and energy to continue the program that eventually resulted in a long-term, healthy nutritional plan. Her monitoring program may have been elaborate, but it worked. Monitoring can really help you succeed.

———

Let's resume Kate's story.

She developed an effective weight-reduction plan by finding out about healthy carbohydrates and fats, and especially the quantity of food she needed. She also began her daily exercise program.

"What's the best way to monitor my nutrition plan?" Kate asked.

"A computer program is helpful, but any way you can record numbers will work," the nutritionist said. "Start with recording your weight. You may not need to weigh yourself every day, but frequently enough to see a trend; once a week is good."

"What else?"

"Just like we talked about before. Measure your waist circumference at the top of the hips. Measure your percentage of fat. You can also make a note of any symptoms you may have. If available, you can monitor your blood pressure and blood sugar."

Over time, Kate reached her healthy weight and a healthy fat-percentage level. The monitoring program was helpful because the positives gave her confidence to continue the plan and the negatives helped her discuss the plan with the nutritionist to get back on track.

During one of her visits, Kate told the nutritionist, "I'm confused about two of our friends who used the three nutrition monitors. Both continued to gain weight."

"Send them over. We'll talk," the nutritionist said.

Phil, a family friend, met with the nutritionist. "What's your eating schedule?" the nutritionist asked.

"Oh, it's really simple. I eat one meal each night," Phil said.

"That could be a problem," the nutritionist said.

"What'd you mean? Someone told me it'd work and it made sense. I don't eat anything all day. You'd have to lose weight that way."

"The body has a natural biorhythm for eating," the nutritionist said. "Three meals are usually best. Eating one large meal at night means the extra food that's not turned into energy is turned into fat."

"Oops," Phil said. "I hadn't thought of that, and I was eating a huge amount during that one meal."

Phil changed to three meals a day, eating the right types of foods, but his weight did not decrease.

"It didn't work," Phil said to the nutritionist during his next visit.

"Try this. Write down what you eat for a few days—not only the names of foods but the quantity."

Phil returned a week later. "There's the answer," Phil and the nutritionist said simultaneously as they reviewed the information.

"It's a quantity problem," Phil said. "It's off the chart. It looks like I keep having second helpings at night and even for lunch on some days." He was subconsciously eating two helpings and didn't realize it until he wrote it down.

"You need to eat to your energy level," the nutritionist said.

"What'd you mean?"

"You can eat until you're Thanksgiving-full or you can eat to your energy level. Ancient gurus knew they needed just enough food to have a feeling of increased energy. After that, it's a feeling of losing energy and being full."

"So this has been known for centuries?"

"Yup, and at first it's difficult because your stomach is not filled up and has not triggered the fullness reflex. But train your mind. Use the feeling that you've gained energy at its peak and additional food will decrease energy. It's a subtle but true feeling that you can learn over time."

"I've never heard of it, but it sounds good," Phil said. "I'll try it."

The nutritionist was right. Phil was able to experience the feeling and learned to make it a routine. The quantity of food decreased to about half the previous amount. It was hard work at first because there was no feeling of being filled up, but Phil persisted and soon returned to a healthy weight for him.

Another of Kate's friends, Anna, visited the nutritionist.

"You've been gaining weight, and you've been eating the right types of foods and the right quantities. Do you have any specific measurements?" the nutritionist asked.

"Yes, I've been measuring my weight and waist circumference."

"What'd they show?" the nutritionist asked.

"The weight circumference was increasing faster than anything else," Anna said. "I also monitored my feelings and any new symptoms."

"Did anything show up?"

"Yes. My face was getting round, which I thought was strange because I always had an angular face. I even developed stretch marks around my middle, and I definitely was not pregnant. My skin seemed fragile; red and purple splotches appeared out of nowhere."

"That's quite a collection of findings. Anything else?"

"I even developed acne, which I never had, and I'm really tired all of the time. I'm embarrassed, but I even have facial hair."

"These symptoms sound like you're taking corticosteroid medicine like prednisone," the nutritionist said.

"No, I'm not taking any medication or supplements."

"We need to send you for a cortisol suppression test to see if you're producing excess cortisol."

During the next visit, the doctor and nutritionist talked to Anna about the test results and diagnosis. The test showed a very high cortisol level. This could mean an adrenal gland tumor secreting the cortisol, a pituitary tumor near the brain stem secreting a cortisol-stimulating hormone, or even a very rare cancer someplace in the body secreting cortisol.

"That's really scary," Anna said. "Could I die from this?"

"One step at a time," the doctor said. "Let's obtain an abdominal computerized (CT) scan, because a tumor in one of the adrenal glands is the most likely cause."

The scan confirmed a left-sided adrenal tumor. These are usually benign tumors like adenomas, which mean they're not cancers that spread, but they continue to grow and produce increasing amounts of cortisol, eventually leading to multiple organ failure.

They reviewed the treatment options. The best option for her was surgical removal of the tumor. She underwent the surgery without difficulty. It was an adenoma located in the adrenal gland that secreted the excessive cortisol. She was cured.

She had been eating the right types of food and the right quantity before the tumor, so she quickly returned to her healthy weight after the surgery. Anna's monitors resulted in a quick diagnosis and successful treatment

———

Monitoring your nutritional status can result in all types of helpful information. The positives tell you that you are on the right path. The negatives tell you to explore new issues. We'll discuss creating an environment in which to heal in the next chapter, and conclude Kate's story.

Create a Healing Environment:
Healthful Eating, Exercising, Sleeping

How can anyone be healed who is dangerously overweight and has diabetes, hypertension, and cardiovascular disease?

Zoe has the answer. She took antidiabetic pills, antihypertensive pills, and heart pills every day, yet she was healed.

Overweight, diabetes, hypertension, heart problems, taking pills every day—how could Zoe claim to be healed? Because she used the power of her own words and thoughts. She used the combined energy of her mind and body. And she was following her nutritional management plan. She was seeing gradual weight loss and improvement in her diabetes and high blood pressure.

The first four steps in nutrition management involve learning, diagnostic testing, treatment, and monitoring. The fifth step is to create a healing environment by combining the physical attributes of the body and the powerful influence of the mind. The body has a remarkable ability to heal itself.

There are three physical components and five elements related to the mind. You've learned about nutrition, which is the first of the three physical components. The others are exercise and sleep.

Exercise is the most amazing thing you can do for yourself. It can save your life.

———

Sterling, 78, believed he had no need to own an automobile, a decision he made at age 25 while studying in England. He walked everywhere, every day, to every place. He gradually developed a routine that included a 45-minute walk each morning, no matter where he was. At age 74, he faced a major surgical emergency that would have resulted in a fatal outcome for a weak person, but he survived with strength, returning to his active life within a few days. This is a powerful lesson. His idiosyncratic thinking 50 years ago of having no use for an automobile led him to daily walks that saved his life.

———

You can start your exercise program with something you like—walking, running, swimming, or an exercise club. Begin slowly; ten minutes every other day, and increase duration and frequency to 20 minutes every day for health benefits, and increase it to 45 minutes to one hour three to five times weeks for really powerful benefits like stress relief and a feeling of strength and well-being.

Join a workout facility and mix it up—cross-training, body pump or Zumba dance fitness classes, spinning, weights, machines, and workouts with a trainer. For individual workouts, it's helpful to use a personal trainer at first to design a program for you and to learn the right way of doing the exercises so you'll use all muscle groups and avoid hurting yourself. Most facilities have introductory sessions.

If you have an underlying chronic medical disorder, cardiac or pulmonary rehabilitation programs are excellent ways to begin exercising because you're in a protected environment. Your heart rate and oxygen will be monitored. You'll be surprised when you discover how much exercise you can do. You'll be taught about strength training exercises too. Best of all, you'll learn an exercise program that you can continue at home or at a workout facility.

Strength training needs to be part of your exercise program because it can delay loss of lean body mass. Each decade of aging results in loss of functional lean muscle mass, and this process accelerates after age 65. It decreases the basal metabolic rate so fewer calories are needed, but people usually continue to consume the same number of calories as they age, which results in weight gain.

A sedentary lifestyle can result in the loss of functional lean body mass. You need to include muscle strengthening as part of your workout. A personal trainer can develop a personalized program that will not result in unwanted bulky muscles.

You'll notice short-term effects from an exercise program after the first session, while long-term effects are apparent after three to six months. Full conditioning returns after about three years, at which point you will feel that you are in as good or better shape than you've ever been. Exercise is a powerful way to ignite your latent energy system, creating positive energy that can help you achieve nutrition management.

So the first two traditional components in creating a healing environment include nutrition and exercise. Sleep is the third. Eight hours of sleep is required for a healthy body and mind. Most people just don't get enough sleep.

Take the five-minute sleep test. Sit in a chair in a quiet room. If you fall asleep within five minutes, you will have flunked the test. This might be only an isolated result, or it may mean that you are chronically sleep-deprived, which causes neural behavioral changes and cardiovascular complications. In addition, you could fall asleep while with family and friends, during an important meeting at work, or while driving.

A healthy sleep-hygiene program includes not allowing yourself to fall asleep watching television before you go to bed, not eating or eating little within three hours before you go to bed, and going to sleep and waking up at regular times.

A brief nap in the afternoon may be effective for some individuals, but sleeping one to two hours just before you go to bed will have devastating results. You'll be awake for hours and will toss and turn throughout the night.

Sometimes a relaxation technique such as yoga or a deep-breathing exercise can be helpful before you go to bed. Sleeping pills are not needed if you have a successful sleep-hygiene program. Managing sleep successfully can have a profound impact on the creation of an environment in which to heal.

———

Now that we've covered the three traditional physical components, it's time to learn about utilizing the mind for nutritional management.

First, use a positive approach. You can manage your nutrition. You're in charge. You'll follow your nutrition plan, you'll exercise, and you'll develop a beneficial sleep schedule.

———

Candice was angry. She had been trying to lose weight for 12 years.

"I can't do this," she thought to herself. "I'm mad at the doctors because they can't help me. The nutritionist is really nice, but it's too much work. I hate to exercise. The diets are way too complicated. I don't want to work at it. The pills are too dangerous. I just want to lose weight."

Candice searched the internet for an easy answer. She found only the information that would entrench her negative thinking, until something finally jolted her. Her mind was the solution. If she didn't do something soon, she would develop life-threatening complications.

"I have to change my attitude," she thought. "I can create a plan that will work for me, and because I developed the plan, I *will* be able to follow it."

Candice talked to her nutritionist. She had many conditions and requirements, but the nutritionist listened patiently, and the two of them developed a plan that was perfect for her. It took time, but during the next three years, Candice returned to her healthy weight and developed a flexible plan that allowed her to maintain her healthy weight.

———

Confidence can be a powerful source of energy, so you should remember to have intense confidence in yourself and everyone else.

Second, use visualization. Visualize yourself at your perfect weight and appearance. You can use this mental imaging daily or whenever you think about it.

———

Parker tried visualization as he attempted to lose weight. After eating a gallon of ice cream every night for an extended period, he was carrying an extra 100 pounds of fat. The weight was dangerous in itself, but the excessive saturated fats in the ice cream were depositing fatty plaques on the walls of his coronary arteries at a life-threatening pace. This was especially true for the anterior descending coronary artery that leads down the center of the heart, which is referred to as the "widow maker" because total blockage there will cause an instant fatal heart attack.

So at night, Parker used visualization. In his mind, he saw himself going to the freezer to pick out his favorite ice cream, taking off the lid, and filling a huge bowl with the ice cream. He added peanut butter cups, sprinkles, nuts, and a tower of whipped cream topped with three cherries. In his mind, he had a big bite with everything in it. It tasted wonderful. He had another bite and another. He enjoyed every second, and with each bite he paused to enjoy the pleasure. After a few minutes of this, he stopped. He had made it through the first night without ice cream! Visualization can have a powerful effect on the body.

———

Another way to use visualization is for a sudden food craving. If you have an overwhelming craving for a specific food, visualize it. If it seems appealing, go ahead and eat it. If it doesn't, you're not really hungry. Find a distraction and eat later.

A third way to use the mind for nutrition management is to have compassion for yourself. You're perfect. It's the extra weight, or the diabetes, or the high blood pressure that needs to be eliminated. Be good to yourself.

Fourth, use controlled breathing. This can help you regain calmness and a positive attitude toward nutrition management. There are two helpful methods.

Try belly breathing. It's opposite from your usual breathing routine. Put your hand on your stomach and breathe in. Instead of having your hand move downward when you breathe in, make your hand move upward. After that, blow out your breath moving your hand downward. You only need two or three of these belly breaths. It works. Try this when you find yourself stressed or nervous.

You can utilize the equal-in and equal-out breath technique. Concentrate on breathing in the same amount as breathing out and very smoothly—50% in and 50% out—for several minutes. You will be calmer after a few of these equal breaths.

Fifth, persistence is fundamental for these mind techniques. The techniques are subtle. They take time. You need to train your mind.

Learn to use all of your brain-wave activity, not just the standard waking, 14-cycle-per-second, beta brain-wave frequency. Learn to use the slower and powerful, ten-cycle-per-second, alpha brain waves for creativity, and the slow seven-cycle-per-second, theta brain waves for healing. You can learn to recognize and use these alpha and theta brainwaves with meditation at first, and later, by recall with your mind.

For advanced brainwave consideration, go with the bosons. They're the subatomic pure energy particles from quantum physics that are a gregarious group, each identical, that travel throughout the universe. Join them for a ride using your creative alpha brainwaves and healing theta brainwaves for relaxation and exploration.

Over and over, replace negative thoughts and actions with these mind-management thoughts. Dismay and hopelessness are powerful emotional feelings that are sometimes uncontrollable and weaken the mind, especially when you're trying to lose weight. They can trap you because they generate sympathy for yourself and from others. Don't fight these feelings. Let them occur, but replace them with neutral or positive thoughts as quickly as possible. They must be replaced with strength, resolve, and persistence, which lead to increased energy for nutrition management.

———

Kate had learned as much as she could about nutrition and had formulated an excellent management plan. Her son did well and her two friends solved their weight-gain problems.

As part of her plan, Kate wanted to create a healing environment.

"What'd you mean by creating a healing environment?" Kate asked the doctor.

"There are examples everywhere," the doctor said. "People can have incurable diseases with potential life-threatening events every day, yet they're healed. Being healed is in the mind."

"I never thought of that," Kate said. "I should be able to do this."

"There are three traditional physical components and several mind-related components," the doctor said.

"You're following two of the three physical components with your nutrition management and exercise programs. The third is a healthy sleep schedule."

"Several years ago," Kate said, "I had heard about the need for eight hours of sleep and developed a great program. I always go to bed at the same time each night and wake up eight hours later. For me, that's 10:00 at night and waking at 6:00 in the morning. I don't eat anything after 7:00 at night. If I'm tired, I take a nap in the middle of the day and don't fall asleep watching television in the evening."

"Excellent. Congratul ations," the doctor said. "You have a phenomenal program.

"There are mind-management factors that can be helpful. Your son, Craig, talked about it. Approach the nutritional problem in a positive way. You *can* do this. As soon as you think that you'll fail or you can never do this, stop these thoughts as fast as you can and return to the thinking of knowing that you're in charge."

"You're right," Kate said. "Craig had that one figured out. What else?"

"Visualization can be effective for people losing weight. Some people tape a picture of themselves on the mirror to remind them of what they could be. Others use a picture of someone they like who is slim."

"I might try that," Kate said.

"It may sound strange, but have compassion for your body in its overweight state, because it's perfect. The extra pounds are the issue, and they can be taken off."

"That's a little strange, but I'll remember it," Kate said.

"Controlled breathing can be helpful to reduce stress," the doctor said. "Use a few abdominal breaths."

"I remember those during the pregnancy classes with my husband," Kate said. "Is that what you mean?"

"Yes, put your hand on your stomach. Breathe in moving your hand up instead of down. It triggers a calming reflex. Try it with me."

Kate put her hand on her lower abdomen, breathed in, and couldn't do it at first, but after two or three times, she did three or four breaths.

"It's a miracle!" she exclaimed. "It really works."

"If you're stressed out before eating, be sure to take three or four of these belly breaths before eating," the doctor said. "Your digestive system will be grateful and work more efficiently."

"Sounds good. Anything else?"

"You can also use the equal-breath technique, which means you breathe in the same amount that you breathe out, 50% in and 50% out. As you do this, you also need to concentrate on making the in-breath and out-breath very smooth. Do this for a few minutes. It has a healthy and calming effect."

This is the end of Kate's story. She's a hero because she completely resolved her weight-related problem on a long-term basis despite the tremendous obstacles that developed along the way. She also helped other people with their nutritional issues.

The five steps can lead to success. Kate learned everything she could about nutrition. She understood the diagnostic process and knew the treatment options. She had a good monitoring system and she developed a healing environment.

———

You can manage your nutrition. You know the five-step approach.

Learn everything you can about nutrition and keep learning. Understand the diagnostic process. Know the treatment options and keep current as new developments continue to emerge. Monitor your nutrition because the information will lead to successful management. Continue to create an environment in which to heal using mind-body connections.

You're in charge of your nutrition.

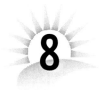

Quick Facts and Rules to Live By

Eat the highest quality of foods that you can buy,
and in the right amount.

Learn to eat to your high-energy level, not your
over-stuffed, low-energy level.

Good carbs: Vegetables, legumes, whole grains, and fiber.

Learn about thresholds for carbohydrates.

Avoid low-threshold carbohydrates.

Bad-quantity carbs trigger weight gain and inflammation.

Good fats: Omega-3 fatty acids and unsaturated fats.

Learn about thresholds for fats.

Avoid low-threshold fats.

Bad-quantity fats trigger inflammation.

Eliminate trans fat.

Minimize sugar.

Minimize saturated fats.

Minimize sodium.

Minimize processed foods.

Eat plenty of fiber.

Listen to your belly brain.

Eat sitting down.

Start an exercise program.

Get eight hours of regular sleep—same time to bed
and same time to rise.

Approach your nutrition challenge in a positive way.

———

You are in charge.

You can manage your nutrition.

You can do this better than anyone else.

Your chance of success is unlimited.

About the Author

Dr. Gary Epler is a clinician, author, and educator. He has written the critically acclaimed, personalized health book, "You're the Boss: Manage Your Disease." He obtained his medical degree from Tulane University in New Orleans and his master's degree in public health from Harvard University in Boston.

Recognized yearly from 1994 to 2012 in "The Best Doctors in America," Dr. Epler is a pulmonary consultant at Brigham and Women's Hospital and Dana-Farber Cancer Institute in Boston, as well as a clinical associate professor of medicine at Harvard Medical School. For 15 years, he chaired the Department of Medicine at New England Baptist Hospital in Boston.

This is Dr. Epler's fourth book in the "You're the Boss" series, written for people everywhere so that they can easily learn how to manage their health and diseases.

While exploring Colombia and the Amazon jungle as a medical student, Dr. Epler discovered the missing cercaria stage of the lung fluke. Later, he probed the nutritional needs of people living in the lower Sahara region of Africa, and he managed the tuberculosis refugee program in Southeast Asia.

Dr. Epler is world-renowned for describing the lung disorder, bronchiolitis obliterans organizing pneumonia, or BOOP, which spurred international research and study. In the 1990s, he developed an interactive website about BOOP, idiopathic pulmonary fibrosis, or IPF, and sarcoidosis for patients and their families.

In addition to conducting clinical and research work, Dr. Epler strives to educate. He became editor-in-chief of an internet-based educational program in critical care and pulmonary medicine offered by the American College of Chest Physicians. *Business Week* acclaimed him for his development of e-health educational programs that enable patients to manage their health and diseases.

Dr. Epler was recognized as one of Boston Magazine's "2007 Top Doctors in Town." He has received numerous teaching awards. He has published books about occupational lung diseases and bronchiolar diseases. He has written more than 100 scientific articles and presented some 350 lectures and seminars worldwide. He is a frequent guest on radio and television shows.

Active in his community, Dr. Epler has coached soccer, hockey, and basketball, and he recently coached a college-club baseball team. He lives near Boston with his wife, Joan, and their two sons.

Visit www.eplerhealth.com for updated information about personalized health and for help managing your nutrition.